Win at
the gym

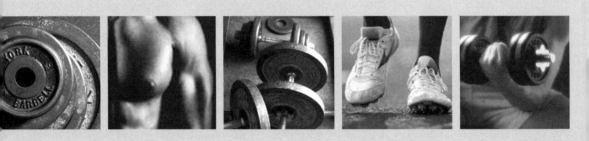

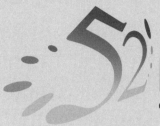

brilliantideas

one good idea can change your life...

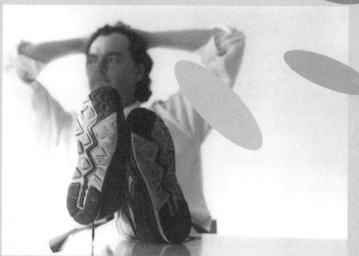

Win at the gym

Steve Shipside

CAREFUL NOW...

Before beginning any exercise programme, it is advisable to obtain the approval and recommendations of your doctor. While you are following any exercise programme, it is advisable to visit your doctor for periodic monitoring.

Mention of specific companies in this book does not necessarily imply endorsement by the publisher, nor does it imply that those companies endorse the book.

Know your limits and don't take risks beyond your level of experience or ability. It's your body, and it's up to you to take responsibility for your own safety and progress. Fix your own goals and focus on your own workout – not what other people are doing. Attempting to compete without knowing what you're doing is the fast track to coming a cropper. There's no point getting the fitness bug only to crock yourself and end up spectating sulkily from the sidelines.

Any form of exercise activity poses potential health risks. Inactivity, on the other hand, makes health risks a certainty.

Copyright © The Infinite Ideas Company Limited, 2004

The right of Steve Shipside to be identified as the author of this book has been asserted in accordance with the Copyright, Designs and Patents Act 1988

First published in 2004 by
The Infinite Ideas Company Limited
Belsyre Court
57 Woodstock Road
Oxford
OX2 6HJ
United Kingdom
www.infideas.com

CIP catalogue records for this book are available from the British Library and the US Library of Congress.

ISBN 1-904902-00-6

Designed and typeset by Baseline Arts Ltd, Oxford
Printed and bound by TJ International, Cornwall

Brilliant ideas...

Looking the part (as opposed to looking like a part) is probably the least of your concerns but proper gym wear can make all the difference between a good session and an afternoon in A&E.

Warming up is a bit like going regularly to the dentist. We all know we should, we all pay lip service to the benefits, we all skip it as often as we can.

When you've just done a hard session the temptation is to hit the shower/pub as soon as possible. The success of your next session is at stake, however, if you don't take the time to cool down.

You've been exercising for some time so you're fitter, yes? But how fit? How hard are you working? How do you know if you're in the fat-burning zone or working at your threshold?

If some is good, then more must be better, right? If it's virtuous to go to the gym three times a week, then five times must make me something of a saint, no? No.

Brilliant features

Each chapter of this book is designed to provide you with an inspirational idea that you can read quickly and put into practice straight away.

Throughout you'll find four features that will help you to get right to the heart of the idea:

- *Try another idea* If this idea looks like a life-changer then there's no time to lose. *Try another idea* will point you straight to a related tip to expand and enhance the first.

- *Here's an idea for you* Give it a go – right here, right now – and get an idea of how well you're doing so far.

- *Defining ideas* Words of wisdom from masters and mistresses of the art, plus some interesting hangers-on.

- *How did it go?* If at first you do succeed try to hide your amazement. If, on the other hand, you don't this is where you'll find a Q and A that highlights common problems and how to get over them.

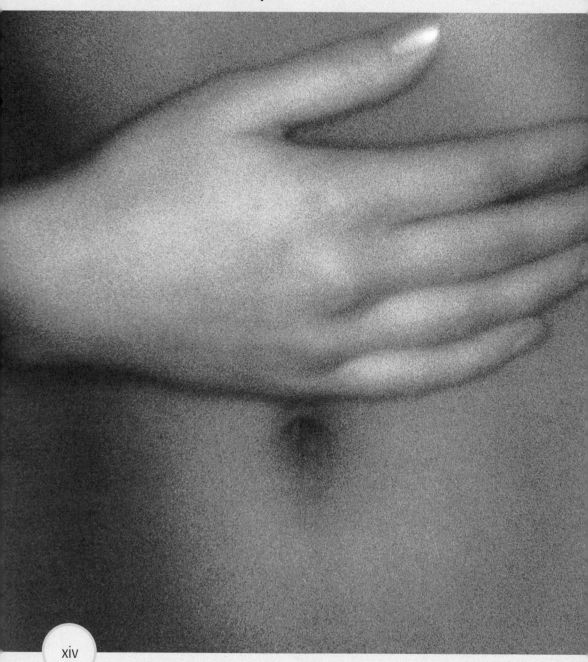

Introduction

Ask yourself the following...
Are you keen to lose weight?
Want to tone up that body?
Looking for stamina and health gains?
Bored witless in the gym?

So you've got over the hurdle of hauling yourself off the couch and down to the gym. Great.

You've located the lockers, you know how to use at least half the buttons on the treadmill, and you've embarked on an on–off fling with a couple of classes and a weight machine or two. But now the initial wave of enthusiasm is some way behind you, and you're not entirely sure you're getting anywhere. If you're honest the Beast of Boredom is snapping at your ankles as you exercise and your gym routine is getting, well, routine.

Which is where this book comes in. It's not written by a sporting superstar or professional athlete. The author is not even a natural gym rat, in fact on bad mornings he barely makes the grade as a mammal.

It's written by an ordinary guy with a day job and Better Things To Do (looking out the window, making paperclip daisy chains, going to the pub...) who embarked on a fitness journey that saw him go from overweight keyboard jockey to extreme triathlete. He still doesn't know what it feels like to stand on the winner's podium, but there is nothing he can't tell you about gym boredom. In order to keep training, year in, year out, he has had to dig deep into the secrets of spicing up those gym sessions. Professional athletes, running partners, personal trainers – all the people he's ever exercised with have been frisked, pick-pocketed or brutally mugged for their ideas on how to keep up the gym momentum. You're holding the results in your hand right now.

Here's how to set goals, avoid burn out and measure your progress. How to use those really obscure machines that lurk menacingly in the corner of the weights room. How to banish boredom on the stationary bike and defeat the tedium of treadmill time. You'll find ideas for the most entertaining classes, and details of those subtle tweaks that turn ordinary moves into torture, or that take the pain away. However unlikely it may sound, you'll find yourself having fun as you get fit.

It's intended for men and for women, for those looking to build strength as much as those hoping to burn blubber, for improvers at every level from the seriously grudging, to the wildly overambitious. Stick with it and you will become an indoor triathlete, learn your marathon target time, shimmy yourself svelte and fall off objects you don't even know the name of yet. Thrill to tales of derring-do on the stepper, gasp at scenes of torture on the Roman chair, giggle yourself silly at words like 'fartlek'. Then do it all yourself in your own time and feel the difference.

There *is* gain without pain, you can win in the gym, and you don't have to wear legwarmers. Promise.

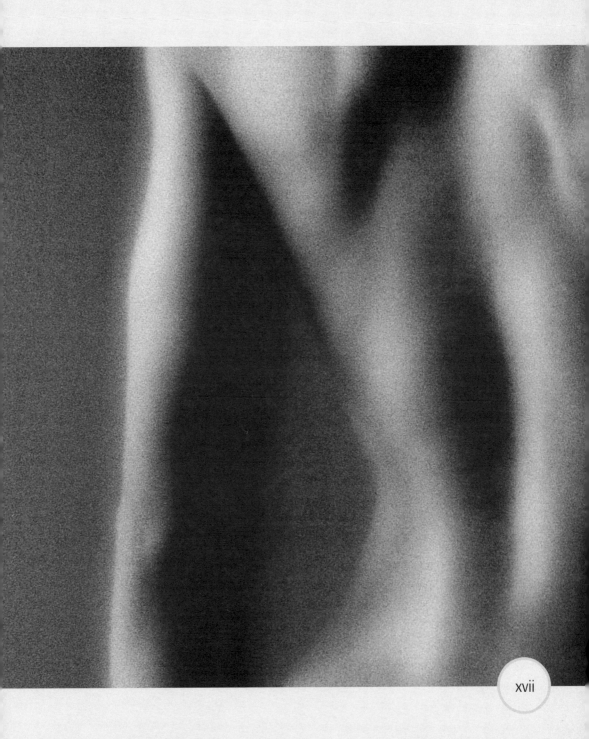

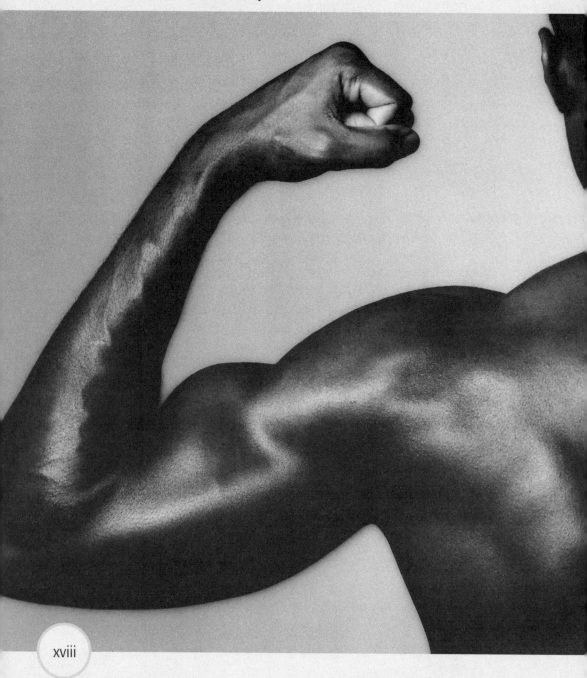

1

Looking the part

Looking the part (as opposed to looking like a part) is probably the least of your concerns but proper gym wear can make all the difference between a good session and an afternoon in A&E.

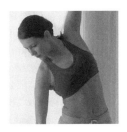

Let's get one thing straight from the start – this idea has nothing to do with fashion.

No area of human endeavour has produced more ludicrous outfits than the fitness business (OK, there's ballroom dancing and golf...). A quick look around any gym will reveal at least a couple of lurid skin-tight nightmares that any self-respecting 70s glam rocker would have turned down as too showy. Fashion gets left behind in the locker, but function, ah now that's another story. When it comes to function the choice between good and bad gear can mean the difference between performing at your peak or winding up in hospital. Read on and rate the contents of *your* gym bag.

KEEPING YOUR FEET ON THE GROUND

Shoes are the make-or-break item in your gym bag, but most people choose them on either price or brand without a thought to what they're actually going to do. Most 'sports' shoes have no right to be in a gym because they're completely unsuitable and won't protect you.

Here's an idea for you...

You can get an idea of whether you're a pronator or supinator simply by looking at the underside of your current shoes and checking the wear pattern. Most of us wear down more on one side of the heel than the other. The way they've worn will tell even more to a shoe specialist, so remember to take your old gym shoes with you when you go to the shop to get advice on a new pair.

Running shoes

What could be simpler than left foot, right foot, repeat? Except that the forces on your body when you run are phenomenal. The entire weight of your bounding body comes crashing down on one small part of your foot. It's only common sense to provide padding at that point but it turns out we all run in different ways and one of the key differences is the way our feet take the shock. To the experts that's called pronation.

With a neutral footfall the first point of impact is the heel. Then the sole of the foot is planted, and the force rolls up toward the ball. Finally you spring off your toes. Loading the heel and the ball with shock absorbers looks like good sense. Or would do if any of us had a truly neutral footfall.

Most of us *overpronate* to a certain degree: our foot lands on the outside edge of the heel and rolls inwards as the weight is shifted to the ball and off again. There's nothing wrong with that, but clearly a well-designed shoe for an overpronator will cushion the outside edge of the foot. And just to make things more awkward, some people do just the opposite and *oversupinate* – they roll their feet outwards. As if that wasn't enough some of us have an unusually strong heelstrike, and some of us strike on the ball of the foot. Each different way of running requires a different design of shoe to minimise the impact. If you overpronate or oversupinate a lot you may even need what are called stability shoes to help balance your biomechanics.

So if you just pick up a pair of shoes on the basis of the colour or the logo you will be doing yourself no favours when it comes to the hard impact of running. There will always be someone who hammers away on the treadmill in nothing but a holed pair of green-flash tennis shoes, but as they get older they will also be the experts on overuse injuries, shin splints and knackered knees.

If you want to make sure you're all kitted up then think about your music – see IDEA 6, *Gettin' jiggy in the gym*.

Try another idea...

There's only one answer. Get thee to a specialist running shop where someone can see you run and suggest shoes to suit you. My favourite shop videos your feet as you run and then talks you through the tape. Some shops have treadmills where you can try out shoes, and all of them have a street outside so there's no excuse for them trying to sell you a shoe if they haven't seen you run in it. A proper fit is key to getting fit. Wear the wrong shoes, with the wrong degree of cushioning, and you're increasing the risk of injury.

Cross-trainers

Running shoes are great for running – but running, while very high impact, is just one kind of motion. Unless you're a very unusual runner indeed your feet will always be moving forwards, whereas the moment you indulge in martial arts, step or just about any other

'If you can't fly, then run. If you can't run, then walk. If you can't walk, then crawl. But whatever you do, keep moving.'
MARTIN LUTHER KING, JR

Defining idea...

training you will start moving sideways, jumping and changing direction suddenly. Now your foot needs lateral cushioning and probably some ankle protection. Enter the cross-trainer. If you fight shy of the treadmill but can't resist those step classes, then you'd do better to get a dedicated cross-trainer. The golden rule is to buy the shoe to suit the job it's going to do, not to suit the suits in the marketing department.

SLICK WICKING

That baggy cotton T-shirt may feel just great, but cotton worn next to the skin is not the best for the roaring gym beastie you are about to become. Work out and you will sweat. Sweat in cotton and your clothes will soon be sporting large, cold, damp patches. For your own comfort and performance, switch to a wicking fabric. Wicking clothes are modern synthetics (careful with them in the wash) that wick sweat away by spreading it rapidly through their fibres where it more readily evaporates. That cools you down in the process. Nike introduced the wicking revolution with a fabric called Dri-Fit but these days every single brand has much the same thing under a different name.

BE IN CONTROL OF THE BOUNCE

Seriously good sports bras are invaluable and for the larger lady that will mean something with a lot more support than a crop top from Sweaty Betty. Try the Less Bounce site (www.lessbounce.co.uk) or SportsBras (www.sportsbras.co.uk).

NO-NOS

No jewellery – please. I don't know how he did it but I can still remember seeing a lad who managed to get his chunky ID bracelet caught in the (moving) seat of the rower he was sitting in. Everyone was so fascinated it was ages before anyone offered to help.

Q   **I went to a specialist running shop and it turns out that I have very wide feet. Is that a problem?**

How did it go?

A   *It can be if you squeeze them into narrow trainers. Even if it doesn't seem uncomfortable your foot will try and bust out through the walls of the trainer which reduces their ability to protect your precious plates of meat. Certain specialist running shoe makers do six widths or more per size. Ask in a good running shop.*

Q   **I've seen people wearing plastic waterproof tops and trousers in the gym to help 'sweat' weight off. Does it work?**

A   *Nope. As well as being plain nasty the 'sweating' weight off approach doesn't get rid of fat. It just makes you lose water. As a result of their extra sweatiness the people in the bin bag outfits will weigh less after the session, but unless they want to be dangerously dehydrated they will have to replace all that lost fluid a.s.a.p. It's true that boxers do it, but that's just to get under a certain weight at the moment of weigh in.*

Q   **Do I need both running shoes and cross-trainers?**

A   *Cross-trainers are all-rounders. If you're serious about running you will need running shoes. If you only venture onto the treadmill for a mile or two a week at gentle pace, then cross-trainers will do you fine – for now.*

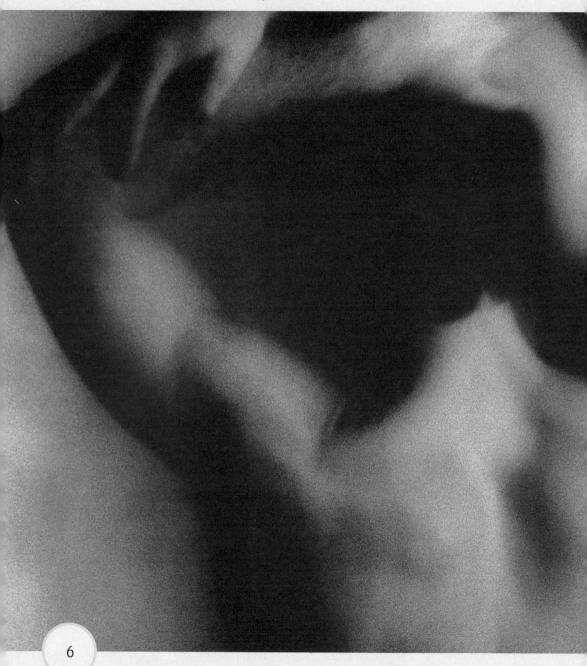

2

Turning up the heat

Warming up is a bit like going regularly to the dentist. We all know we should, we all pay lip service to the benefits, we all skip it as often as we can.

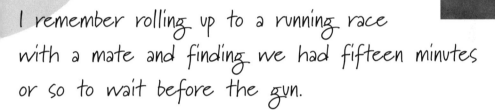

I remember rolling up to a running race with a mate and finding we had fifteen minutes or so to wait before the gun.

We both stood there and looked at the handful of people who were jogging up and down to warm up. 'Shall we, er...?' I ventured. My mate's icy look stopped me dead. The same thought went through both of our minds – with a long-distance race ahead of us who wanted to run a single step more? We fell silent. Me, my mate and several thousand equally stationary 'athletes' went back to watching those noble few doing their warm-ups.

You know you should warm up. You know in your heart of hearts that it reduces the risk of injury and increases your performance. But the chances are that you don't, or at best you grudgingly spend a token minute or so throwing yourself around a bit. At the risk of sounding like your mum, here's why you should do it properly.

Warming up can mean pretty much any moderate exercise that raises the pulse gradually. Even something as simple as a couple of minutes running on the spot will suffice. The purpose of a simple warm-up is also to raise the body temperature and psychologically prepare for the session ahead. That increase in temperature serves

Getting to the gym can be made into part of your workout routine if you treat it as a warm-up. If you drive to the gym, then park further away and walk the last five minutes. If you take a bus or tube, then get off at the stop before. If you walk briskly and change fast, then your pulse and body temperature should still be above normal and you should be more ready for action.

several purposes. Increasing the temperature increases the elasticity of muscle, so reducing the risk of tearing or straining it. It also increases the metabolic rate of cells and the readiness of the nervous system.

Prior to a race or a serious session it is commonly recommended that you warm up for 10–30 minutes. Just before a race, you don't see Olympic athletes huddling like penguins. No, they can be spotted bounding around the stadium doing their warm-ups properly.

For the purposes of a gym session, however, most of us are short on time, and less likely to be working at the limits of our ability. Nonetheless there are still some basic warm-up rules to be followed.

However psyched you are it's not a good idea to throw yourself into a hard session. If you're planning on running hard on the treadmill, then warm up first by setting the speed. First walk comfortably, then faster, then find that point where you are striding so fast you want to break into a run and see if you can hold it there for a minute or so. Unlikely as it may seem, you'll almost certainly record a better time over a short run if you first have a 10 or 20 minute warm-up on the treadmill or elliptical trainer. Try it and see how you get on against the clock.

Confusing stretching and warming up is a common, but potentially, costly mistake. Stretching muscles when cold increases the chance of hurting them (see the point about elasticity above) and stretching on its own is unlikely to raise either your pulse or your body temperature. On the other hand it may lead you to think you've warmed up which makes it more likely that you'll throw yourself into a hard session. Try milder stretching after a bit of warm up – for example run gently for a few minutes and then try stretching at the same time with exercises like high stepping (knees up towards chest) and high kicking (heels to bum).

Warm-ups are only part of the picture (and in your heart you know that already) – now turn to IDEA 3, *Cool it*, and read about cool-downs to complete the routine.

Try another idea...

If you can, choose a warm-up that works both upper and lower body. Even sprinters stop and do press-ups in order to increase blood flow and body temperature.

Always aim to do your cardio first before going to the weights room to push metal around.

Never turn up late for classes, skipping the warm-up and plunging straight into the exercises, and where there is a warm-up remember to use it as such. The guys (they're always guys) who load up the weights in BodyPump during the warm-up simply don't understand what it's about and in their hurry to impress each other they are the most likely to pull something.

'If you spend too much time warming up, you'll miss the race. If you don't warm up at all, you may not finish the race.'

Defining idea...

How did
it go? **Q** **What about warming up with a warm shower, or warm clothing – does that help?**

A *Yes it does. So called 'passive' warming up raises the body temperature but it doesn't have the full benefits of an active warm-up – better than nothing but no real substitute.*

Q **Which cardio machines are good for warming up?**

A *In general those that warm up both upper and lower body. Five to ten minutes on the elliptical trainer and the rowing machine should do the job.*

Q **How does warming up prepare me psychologically?**

A *A good warm-up should help you focus on what you're about to do. If you're getting ready to race it's a time to visualise the outcome and think strategy. For the rest of us rolling up at the gym it's a great time to set aside thoughts of work, etc., and prepare for the very different kind of effort ahead of us.*

3
Cool it – cool-downs

When you've just done a hard session the temptation is to hit the shower/pub as soon as possible. The success of your next session is at stake, however, if you don't take the time to cool down.

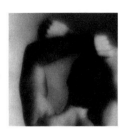

Cool-downs are the flip side of warming up but with a slight twist.

Warm-ups are primarily about ensuring the elasticity of muscle and connective tissue so as to minimise the risk of ripping any of it (see IDEA 2, *Turning up the heat*). Cool-downs, on the other hand, are mainly about getting rid of lactic acid and avoiding blood pooling in the muscles you've just worked so hard to pump full of the stuff.

Coming to an abrupt halt after exercise can also cause cramps, soreness (often due to lactic acid build-up), dizziness or even abnormal strain on the heart.

A good cool-down helps the body return gently to its pre-workout state with breathing and heartbeat falling to normal levels. Keeping moving also allows the blood to be pumped back from the extremities and muscles. As with warm-ups it's important to distinguish cooling down from stretching. Going straight into static stretches isn't going to help your circulation and won't provide the most gentle route back to normality for heart and lungs.

Here's an idea for you... **Cool-downs are your first line of defence against lactic acid build-up and muscle soreness, but you don't have to fight the fight on your own. Massage is a great way of helping your metabolism recover from the effort and trauma of your session. A good massage also helps reinforce the sense of reward and that oh-so-fab feelgood factor.**

Probably the best and simplest cool-down is walking. A good striding motion gradually slowed down to normal pace keeps all the limbs moving rhythmically and lets the lungs catch up. Psychologically it's a great moment to review the session, give yourself a mental pat on the back and come back to the real world. The best time to stretch is after you've done five to ten minutes of cool-down because your muscles will still be at their most flexible. Pretty much every gym class these days has a cool-down section at the end, and there are usually a couple of time-pressed people who see that as their cue to skip off a couple of minutes early. It's understandable but not a good idea. Apart from anything else a proper cool-down contributes massively to the feeling of well-being and smugness after a workout and that feeling is to be encouraged if you want your healthy habit to last.

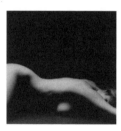

The cool-down is also a great time to reach for that water bottle, and maybe a sports bar or banana to start rehydrating and refuelling. Even if you're only in the gym because you want to lose weight, that post-exercise refuelling session is the key to ensuring your metabolism burns fat reserves rather than trying to hold on to them.

Cool-down is also a great time to check your heart rate, either manually or with a heart rate monitor (see IDEA 4, *Listen to your love muscle*). Your heart rate can drop by 20–40 beats per minute in just a couple of minutes after exercise – and the speed with which it returns to normal is a pretty good indicator of how much fitter you're getting.

Once you've cooled down from your exertions it's time to get stretching to help increase your flexibility (which in turn reduces the chance of injury). Take a look at IDEA 21, *At a stretch*, for more details.

Try another idea...

'Start slow, and taper off.' WALT STACK's advice on marathons. He took his own advice well into his eighties.

Defining idea...

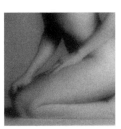

How did it go?

Q **If warming up is so good for my body efficiency, surely there's no problem with me diving into the sauna after a hard work-out?**

A *There can be if you have any heart abnormality. It's always best to cool down gradually for ten minutes or so before risking any sharp rise or fall in temperature – that means icy showers are out too.*

Q **I'm using a heart rate monitor to check myself on cool-downs. What sort of heart rate should I be at?**

A *Only about 50–60 per cent of your max. Since you have a monitor you may also want to note the time it takes for your heart to drop from its exercising maximum down to normal, or to see how far it falls within a set period – say two or three minutes.*

Q **Are there any exercises that need more or less attention to the cool-down?**

A *A cool-down is never going to be a bad thing, but it is true that sometimes it is more important than others. Lactic acid is a by-product of anaerobic exercise so any workout that includes short bursts of maximum effort (such as sprints) will make a cool-down a priority. By contrast, long slow sessions (such as walking) are effectively their own cool-downs.*

4

Listen to your love muscle

You've been exercising for some time so you're fitter, yes? But how fit? How hard are you working? How do you know if you're in the fat-burning zone or working at your threshold?

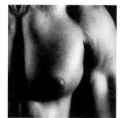

Let your heart show you the way.

THE PROBLEM

We all exercise because we're looking for some kind of benefit – lose weight, look better in a T-shirt, drop a clothes size, dodge that heart attack, live longer to enjoy more time with the grandchildren. The problem is that of these admirable goals some are easier to measure than others. When you fit into smaller clothes, weigh what you did when you were in your twenties or see new muscle definition, then you know you got there. But what of those less obvious but often more crucial goals. How do you know when you are fitter? What is fit anyway? Sooner or later as you plug away on a treadmill or stepper, you'll start to wonder if it's really doing any good. And if you can't tell, then what's the point in giving up your precious time when you could be down the pub.

THE SOLUTION

The answer is to listen to your heart, and the way to do that is to invest in a heart rate monitor. There's nothing that complex about heart monitors – at their simplest you have a transmitter on a chest-strap that broadcasts your heartbeats to a small computer/sports watch on your wrist.

Here's an idea for you...

You can do this with even the simplest monitor, or a stopwatch and two fingers as long as (a) you have the patience and (b) you can find an artery with a pulse. Instead of focusing on zones and percentage of maximum, just do your usual session and then see how long it takes your heart rate to drop to 120 (12 beats within a 10 second period if you're doing it manually). As you get fitter that time will drop, and you may find it becomes more accurate to count how long it takes to get down to 100 beats. Not only can you see your cardiovascular fitness improving week by week, but this can also give you early warning of overtraining or infection as a developing cold can whack that recovery time back up by a 10 or 20 second margin.

HOW DOES IT WORK?

Simple though it sounds, having an accurate idea of your heart rate opens a whole new world of accuracy in training. You can now tell exactly how hard you are working, which is often surprisingly different to how hard you think you are working. By seeing how long it takes for your heart to recover from bursts of exercise you now have access to one of the best indicators of how fit you really are.

IN PRACTICE

The first thing with heart rate monitoring is to establish your maximum heart rate. There's a rule of thumb that 220 minus your age gives your maximum. On that basis a 40 year old would have a maximum heart rate of 180. That's a little imprecise, and there are many other formulae that take account of sex and bodyweight. Because there is this slight variation it's best to follow the instructions that come with your heart monitor.

Once you're at your maximum heart rate, the next step is working out the different training zones. Roughly speaking there are three main training zones: 60–75 per cent of max which is considered easy and often called the 'fat-burning zone', 75–85 per cent of max which is moderate and sometimes referred to as the 'cardio-training zone'; and 85–95 per cent which is giving it some welly and normally only of interest to those going for peak performance and ever-diminishing times.

WHAT THE MONITOR DOES, AND HOW TO CHOOSE ONE

The simplest monitors consist of a stop watch (well you don't want to have two things strapped to your wrist) and will tell you what your rate is. The next step up feature alarms that can be set for zones so, for example, the monitor will beep at you if you get out of the fat-burning zone, or if you drop below a certain level of workload. This is one of the best uses for a monitor and well worth having.

Beyond that level monitors start sprouting all sorts of functions...

- A graphical readout showing a chart of your heartbeat is handy to see how long it takes for your heart to recover after rest.

- A memory of different sessions makes it easy to compare and see your progress.

- Downloadable details are a delight for the number crunchers who like to plot their progress on a spreadsheet.

Try another idea...

Now you can see how hard you're working, try turning to IDEA 8, *Row like Redgrave II*, or IDEA 10, *Run like Radcliffe II*, and try the interval training sessions there but this time with an eye on how hard you are working.

Defining idea...

'My heartbeat is kickin', it's kickin' louder and louder It's getting' deffer and deffer, I'm feelin' prouder and prouder.'
ICE-T, popular vocalist and apparently a man with a keen understanding of the importance of heart rate.

■ 'Shielded' transmitters mean you can workout alongside a partner without their monitor interfering with yours.

■ Calorie counters can be programmed with your physical details to monitor how many calories you burn during the day.

■ Programmable sessions mean you can choose an interval session and never look at your watch again – the monitor beeps at you when you have to slow down/speed up and keeps an eye on how hard you're working.

■ GPS is considered the king of the crop right now – the monitor doesn't just watch your heart, it uses satellite tracking to tell you exactly how far you have run/cycled when you're out doors and what speed you are doing at any moment.

Q   **Why would I need a monitor? I know when I'm giving it some.**

How did it go?

A   *What the pros called 'perceived effort' is a tricky area because very motivated individuals tend to block out discomfort and non-motivated ones tend to exaggerate it. The same level of work could appear easy to one and hellish to another. At the top end of the scale your body releases chemicals that suppress the pain when you're really giving it welly and so you may have difficulty knowing just how hard it is. Your heart, however, won't skip a beat or lie to you.*

Q   **I feel I'm working easily but my heart rate is sky-high. What's going on?**

A   *Are you sure you're not overtraining or coming down with an infection? Either can send your heart rate soaring. Try training at 60–70 per cent of your heart rate for half an hour or more (think of all that fat burning) for a week or two and then go back to your normal efforts. If your heart rate is dangerously high or unpredictable, then see your GP.*

Q   **The monitor manual keeps referring to my RHR. What's this?**

A   *Resting heart rate (RHR) is strictly speaking what level your heart settles down to when you're asleep. Unless you have a partner to help read this off in the night it's usually measured at the moment you wake up. Even so, some people wake up stressed about the day ahead and that can give a slightly high reading. You may get a more accurate level as you wake up covered in newspapers on the sofa this Sunday.*

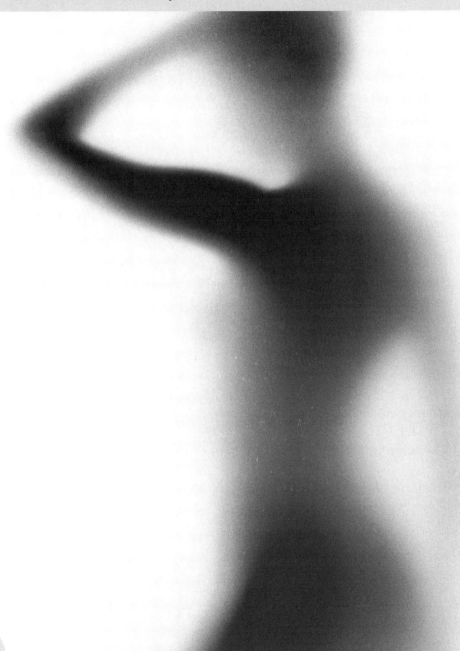

5
Quality versus quantity

If some is good, then more must be better, right? If it's virtuous to go to the gym three times a week, then five times must make me something of a saint, no? No.

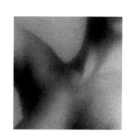

Here's why training smart can often mean training less.

JUNK TRAINING

Just think for a minute about how you count your fitness sessions. Are you a runner clocking up miles? A calorie-burner staring at the dial as the numbers click by? A class-counter aiming to put in three classes a week? Or a clock-watcher ticking off the hours? Maybe you haven't even asked yourself the question yet because you go to the gym pretty much when it's convenient and do some stuff for however long that takes.

Maybe that suits you, but the chances are that if you're reading this book it's because you feel that somehow things could be better, more interesting, more rewarding or more effective.

What happens to many of us is that having started to go to the gym we feel better about ourselves and then a gentle confusion sets in. It seems like being in the gym is what makes us feel good. So we go and try new classes. We may spend an extra half an hour on a machine, particularly something nice and comfy where you can

Here's an idea for you... **Losing weight is all well and good but muscle is denser and thus heavier than fat. If you're strength training while calorie burning you could end up in way better shape but actually weigh more. So forget weight and instead worry about the percentage of your body that consists of fat rather than muscle and bone. How do you do that? Simple: get yourself tested for body fat percentage either at the gym or by buying body composition 'scales' that pass a low-level electrical current through you to find out how much fat you have.**

sit down. Next time we may even take a relaxing read on the exercise bike and come away an hour later feeling that this exercise thing really isn't at all bad. Which is just fine for as long as it works, but this kind of exercise isn't really training, it's more about remaining in a comfort zone. Worse, while it's true that using a machine or going to a class will always achieve some goals (burning calories for example), you need to take a good look at the rest of your life to ensure that you're not then wiping them out afterwards. A lot of people reward themselves for having gone to the gym. That may be as obvious as a face-full of snacks afterwards, or it might be something more insidious like not taking the stairs or driving to the newsagents because, well, you are going to the gym regularly after all. This is the danger of junk training. It doesn't actually do any good in itself, and because it lets you kid yourself you have worked out, you may let things slip elsewhere.

This doesn't mean that the gym always has to be about pain, just that if you don't have a clear goal for each and every visit then you might be better off skipping that session. Similarly if you're not feeling good enough to reach your goal, then why not take the day off and go for it next time instead? Going for quality not quantity works fine for a while, but before long you'll hit a plateau of tiredness, boredom and disappointment.

SO WHAT'S THE ANSWER?

The answer is to draw up some goals, and the means of measuring them. Working out three times a week or spending five hours in the gym is what's called a *process goal* because it focuses on the process not on the actual outcome. If that's all that's getting you to the gym, then you've probably already seen the limitations. Time to move on beyond the process and start setting yourself *outcome goals*. Typical outcome goals tend to be along the lines of:

- Lose weight
- Build bigger arms
- Tighten that bum
- Get back into a size ten
- Get fitter

Speed, endurance, weight and even muscle can all be measured, but what about fitness? How do you know if you are generally fitter? Well there is a way, and that way is to measure your own heartbeats – take a look at IDEA 4, *Listen to your love muscle.*

Try another idea...

It's simple: if it jiggles, it's fat.'
ARNOLD SCHWARZENEGGER

Defining idea...

All of which are admirable in themselves, but a bit vague. If you want results you need to work out how to measure them and give yourself a deadline:

- Build 2 cm of muscle onto the arms by that short break at Easter
- Lose 2 kg before the end of next month
- Get fit enough to run a sub-fifty-minute 10,000 m on a fixed date.

Now you have goals, ways to measure them and deadlines, you can go back to the gym and decide whether you are really achieving something, or just junk training.

How did it go?

Q   **I've decided to lose six kilos this month and am burning 1000 kcals a day on the treadmill to do it. How come I'm tired and getting nowhere?**

A   *Whoah. Goals don't mean unrealistic ones. For a start you're trying to lose more weight than is healthy per week (more than two pounds or a kilo a week and you're pushing it) and you're doing it by way of a routine that only hardened runners will be comfortable with. Set the gate too high and you may lose heart and give up.*

Q   **I'm happy turning in my half hours on the reclining bike? What's wrong with that?**

A   *If you're happy, then good for you. For now. My money says that in the long run, however, you'll either stop going to the gym or come back to this book for more ways to push yourself.*

Q   **I've cut out the junk training and focus just on strength – every day – but I'm getting nowhere. Why can't I seem to make any progress?**

A   *Every day? As in the same thing every day? Mixing and matching is the best way of keeping your body guessing so that it has to keep getting better just to keep up. Try some different training. Remember that you get stronger while you rest, not while you work, so make sure you have at least a day off in between working muscles hard. If you have to work out every day, try alternating muscle groups.*

6

Gettin' jiggy in the gym

Music may or may not be the food of love but it certainly makes the time fly when you're performing the flywheel fandango on rowers or exercise bikes. The only thing is that someone else's choice of music can just as easily put a stick in your (imaginary) spokes.

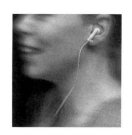

Gyms and music have always gone together, but the results are sometimes less Torvill and Dean, more Laurel and Hardy.

I was once concentrating on my footwork in the treadmill tango when the gym staff decided to put on Leonard Cohen. Ten minutes of gravel-voiced lament about suicide and the whole place was grinding to a halt in a morass of apathy and a desire to drown our sorrows in something a damn site stronger than Lucozade.

People have always liked working out to music, but they often confuse good music with good workout music. If the music is real listening music, music you want to pay attention to, then you may not be paying enough attention to the exercise you're meant to be doing. However attached you may be to a Schubert sonata or humpback whale song you'd be best advised to leave them at home. Good workout music tends to be energetic, rousing and definitely more about beat than about lyrics.

When you record your compilation take note of how long each song is. Next time you're on a cardio machine cover the readout with a towel, shut your eyes and keep going for a set number of songs – five, ten, whatever. Time will pass way faster than when you're watching waiting for the moment you can stop.

Music has always been a hot topic of conversation for athletes online, and particularly among cyclists and triathletes. During the winter many of these boys and girls cycle train on a 'turbo' (a hi-tech version of putting your back wheel up on bricks), and if you think a treadmill is dull, then you should try a turbo. Since turbos are noisy they are often relegated to garages and cellars so the scenery isn't overly pretty either, which is why these people rely on music perhaps more than any others. I remember a poll of what people listened to as they pounded away head-down over the handlebars. Despite the bulk of them being well beyond thirty, the surprise top of the pops were thrash metal and rave culture dance music.

The reason why dance and trance work so well is that they are aimed at people who are off their heads one way or another and aiming to carry on moving to the beat right through the night. You may not like to compare yourself to a nightclub full of teenagers ripped to the gills but there are times when that mindless motion is precisely what you're aiming for.

Which brings us back to the gym. Most gyms have canned music over speakers – which is useless for rhythm since it's half drowned out by the sound of machines. Many have radio stations or TV channels but you'll quickly learn that even 'dance' channels and MTV seem to be about fifty per cent talk. Which isn't what you want as you try to attain that trance-like out-of-body feeling that floats you ever onwards.

BRING YOUR OWN

BYO music is the answer. Don't just use that Steps CD that's lying there but make your own compilation of upbeat energy. Plenty of people make up their favourite party compilations;

Looking for another way to incorporate music into your workout for variety – try IDEA 9, *Run like Radcliffe I: Fartlek.*

Try another idea...

why do so few put the same effort into jazzing up the gym session? Putting together a selection you really want to hear will help put some spice into your next session. Guaranteed.

THE PLAYBACK POSER

Which leaves the question of how to play your personal soundtrack. Tapes have gone the way of the dodo. Think about CDs, MiniDisc, MP3s or hard-drive jukeboxes.

CD Walkmen are cheap and cheerful, but unless you have a good one they can skip. If you weigh anything more than, say, Kylie, then the vibes from your bouncing bod may well send the CD off the machine, let alone cause it

'You are the music while the music lasts.'
T. S. ELIOT, poet and grand master of losing yourself in the groove.

Defining idea...

to skip. Plus, unless you have a computer with a CD burner you may not be able to create your own compilations.

MP3 players have to be loaded up with music via a computer and unless you carry a (small, fiddly, easily-lost) spare memory card you can't then change what you've got at the gym. That said, they are small enough to be worn as jewellery and solid-state so you can play basketball with them and they still won't miss a beat.

MiniDiscs aren't solid-state so they can skip, but most have enough buffer not to in normal use. Much easier than CDs to record to as they don't need a computer and can plug into your hi-fi. If you are using a computer, then make sure you get a 'Net' MiniDisc that can plug into the USB port. It works out much faster than normal recording.

Hard-drive jukeboxes. Think Apple iPod or the Creative Labs' Jukebox Zen. These things are hard drives big enough to hold gigabytes of data which in English means they can hold and play your entire music collection. They can also search for that elusive track in milliseconds and shuffle the tracks to play randomly. For hardcore long session experts the hard-drive jukebox is the Holy Grail.

How did it go?

Q   I have a MiniDisc which I rest on the treadmill/stepper but it still jogs – how do I stop it?

A   *Did it come in a small cloth bag? If not, then get yourself one (or buy a carrying bag from a sports shop) and use a velcro strap to attach it to the machine's handles. If it's hanging off the machine it doesn't pick up so much vibration.*

Q   I lurve ma kickin' music but sometimes have trouble keeping up on the treadmill. Any ideas?

A   *However tempting it is to run to the beat you are risking disaster if you try to match your footfalls to it as it will mean stretching or shortening your stride unnaturally. Try to enjoy the music in your head but let your legs do their own thing – this isn't dancing after all.*

7

Row like Redgrave I: Style points

Strength, stamina and smoothness are the promise of the rowing machine. So why do so many users look less like Steve Redgrave and more like Mr Bean? As with so many things, it's all down to style.

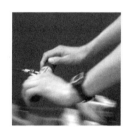

Rowing is right up there with swimming as one of the best all-round exercises you can do — but with the handy difference that you don't have to navigate shrieking ten-year-olds at half term and you're unlikely to end up with a nose full of chlorinated piss.

Done properly, rowing is a great calorie burner, combining weight control with strength development and a cardio workout. It works your legs, your arms, shoulders and back muscles. Do it badly, however, and you end up staggering away from the machine bent over double in those 'ooooh me lumbago' poses beloved of ancient TV sitcoms. So here's the low-down on rowing like Redgrave – how to build strength and stamina with smoothness and precision.

Here's an idea for you...

See the lever on the flywheel that sets the difficulty level? On pretty much all the machines you'll see in the gym it can be set from anywhere between 1 and 10. Pros call it the 'damper', and if you're using a standard air flywheel it lets air in or out. Set it at 1 and it keeps the air trapped in the wheel cage. Since the resistance you feel is the air being turned, and trapped air is already spinning from the last stroke, this gives least resistance. Shove it up to 10 and the air that you've just grunted to spin around is released and replaced with fresh air that you have to get moving again from scratch – hence the extra effort. Not many people know that. In fact few of us really understand resistance levels at all, with the result that the unsure slot the lever down to 1 and most blokes whack it up to 10 in case anyone should think they're not Olympic heroes. Real Olympic heroes tend to go for the feel that is most like a real boat, which according to Terry O'Neill, former Olympic rowing coach, means a level of 3 or 4. Then they concentrate on stroke rate, aiming for about 35 strokes a minute. Next time, instead of thrashing away at the maximum setting, try taking a leaf from the real-life water warriors, and see how long you can keep up the same pace.

BREAKING IT DOWN

Beginners look at the rowing action and see two parts: the pull back, which is the hard bit where they grunt and sweat; and the flop forwards again, which is the easy bit – at least until they put their backs out. Pros, however, break the action down into four distinct movements:

The catch

You're sat on the rower and your feet are safely strapped so you're all ready to unleash the Herculean force of your whole body without your feet flying off so you end up with your ankles wrapped around your ears. It's time for the catch. Slide forward so your shins are vertical, and you have the handle grasped in both hands with your wrists flat and your torso leaning slightly forwards from the hips.

The drive

The powerhouse for this is the legs *and never the arms*. So straighten those legs, pushing hard against the foot rests, and keep the arms straight for the first part of the drive. As your legs straighten out and you are nearing the end of the drive, then your arms start to bend slightly and your upper body comes into play leaning slightly backwards.

The finish

Legs straighten completely, upper body leans lightly backwards, and you pull the handle in towards your stomach just below your rib cage. At the end of the pull your elbows should be tucked in close to your body and behind your back, not sticking out sideways as if you're doing the Birdie Song.

The recovery

First the arms extend forwards, then your upper body leans lightly forward, and your legs bend as you slide smoothly back towards the flywheel down by your feet.

And back to the catch ...

It sounds simple enough, but if you bear the above in mind and take a good look at your fellow gym rowers you'll see that there are plenty of people who snatch at the handle, and try to pull back with their arms. Others end the whole movement still hunched forward or learning backwards, even as they recover. There's always one,

Confident that you've mastered it, smooth and strong all the way? Now bored witless and looking for a goal beyond simply clocking up calorie burn/speed/distances? Great, turn to Idea 8, *Row like Redgrave – II: Revenge of the rowing machine*, for workouts and challenges.

Try another idea...

For an idea of how you can improve your stroke count versus distance, try stroke golf as described in IDEA 8.

Try another idea...

Defining
"idea...

"The guys went off at an unbelievable pace and four hours later they were still going at an unbelievable pace!"
Olympic rowing champion, JONNY SEARLE, commentating on Team MAD's 2004 world indoor record breaking 100,000m team event which saw the ten man team complete the distance in 4:12:46.7, at an average 500m split of 1:15.8. *"Pain is temporary,"* added race organizer, JON GOODALL, a man who, it may be noted, wasn't doing the rowing.

inevitably a bloke, who thinks that they will get the best benefit by flogging themselves to death regardless of form in a triumph of strength over style. Get it right, however, and not only do you reduce soreness and the risk of injury, but you will effortlessly increase both your speed and endurance which in turn means you are more likely to enjoy the challenges of IDEA 8.

Q **Why does the muscle that runs from my neck to my shoulders hurt when I'm rowing?**

How did it go?

A *You may well be tensing up your back and arms. Try relaxing your shoulders as you row and keep your grip on the handle firm but light. Think of all those swashbuckling films where the young hero is taught to hold the sword as if it was alive like a bird in the hand.*

Q **I get tired after only a few minutes. Am I doing something wrong?**

A *It could be that you are using too high a resistance setting, or that you are a little out of shape, but the chances are that your biggest problem is poor form. Check for wastes of energy, like rowing with bent wrists, or reaching too far forward at the catch (so your shins go beyond the vertical).*

Q **I'm catching and driving OK, but why do I get tired in the muscles right across my back?**

A *Sounds like you may be trying to get too much force from the finish, rather than from the drive. Try to get more of your stroke from your thighs, then feel the pull move seamlessly through your upper body and arms. Remember that 'put your back into it' is just an expression.*

Q **My lower back hurts. Am I OK?**

A *If you are getting lower back pains, then you must seek the advice of a sports physician. Back pain is no joke, and while more exercise and stretches may well be the answer you should take the advice of an osteopath, chiropractor or doctor before adding any load to your back.*

33

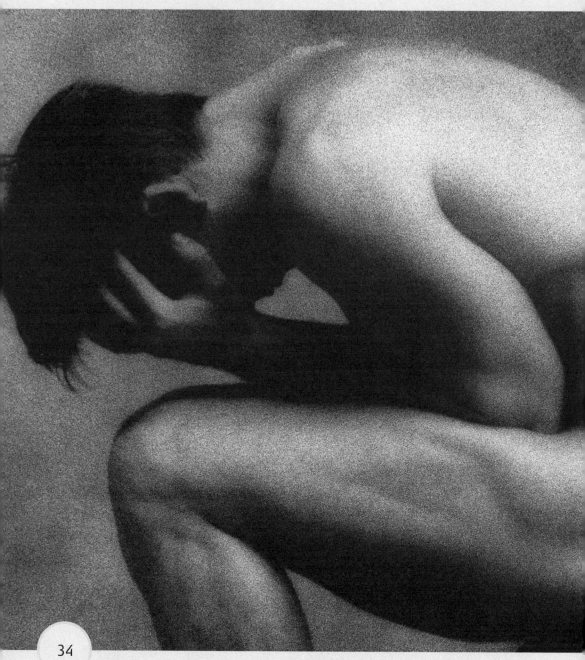

8

Row like Redgrave II: Revenge of the rowing machine

You've mastered the style, you've wiped out those energy-wasting errors and your rowing is now a symphony of power and precision. Great. Now what? Time to step up to your own Olympic challenge.

At their peak Redgrave, Pinsent and co. didn't have to worry about getting bored or going off the boil in the gym.

There were several reasons for this.

First, they had the incentive of being the best in the world, and wanting to stay that way. Second, they had an East German coach bellowing at them if they slowed down for a second. Third, working at the limits of physical endurance they had the bonus excitement of not knowing if they were about to throw up or fall off at any moment.

You and I, on the other hand, probably don't have any of the above – except possibly the third if we go training after a heavy night out. Us mere mortals tend to plateau – we do all right and then hit a point where training doesn't seem to bring

STROKE GOLF
You can do this exercise over any time and at any intensity as a way of working on your style and with it your efficiency. Instead of going for a set speed or distance, just take a sample time – say ten minutes – and complete it at an absolutely fixed stroke rate. The rate can be 18, 24, 30 or whatever you feel comfortable with. At the end of the time note the distance covered. In future sessions keep to exactly the same time, and exactly the same stroke rate, but see if you can increase the distance you cover. If you succeed it's not because you're rowing 'faster' (by upping the number of strokes) but because you're rowing better by getting more power into each stroke.

any benefits. Sure you can try and get through it by training harder, but doing the same thing for longer can get tedious. Going for a gut-busting personal best on speed every time can end up being off-putting, to the point where you dread strapping your feet into the rower and may end up avoiding the gym altogether. Interval training, however, aims to add a little spice to your gym life by mixing and matching on pace, stretching both your speed and your endurance. Whether you're looking for extra power, or simply the motivation to keep on shedding those pounds, interval training can help.

BASICS

First get an idea of your standard pace (and in the process give yourself a yardstick to measure progress) by rowing for 30 minutes without a break. Warm up for five minutes beforehand, and try not to go off too fast at the beginning. Pace yourself so that you have given it all you've got by the end of the half-hour. Not only should that be a nice fat-burning workout for you, but it gives you something to compare with others online at sites like Concept II (www.concept2.co.uk). Once you've got that yardstick, it's time to try one of the following.

PYRAMID ROW

This works much like pyramid sets in weightlifting. Start off gently with a warm-up for a couple of minutes, then start your pyramid. Two minutes fast rowing, followed by two minutes at a pace where you would feel easy enough to chat while rowing (health and safety note: don't chat to strangers while you row – they will hate you, especially if they themselves are breathless). Follow that with three minutes fast, then three minutes easy, then four minutes fast, four minutes easy. That's the pyramid climbed, now for the way back down. After four minutes easy it's back to three minutes fast, then three easy, two fast, then two easy. You get the picture. Feeling hard? Try starting your pyramid at three minutes and going up to five, and if that doesn't get you, then try starting at four and going on to six. The mathematicians among you will have spotted that the effort curve rises sharply each time you notch up the start of your pyramid.

If you're starting to fancy yourself at this mullarky, then it's time to throw down the gauntlet to others. That doesn't have to mean throwing dark looks at the rower next to you; instead try pitting yourself against the times recorded online. Go to the Concept II sites (www.concept2.com) where you can see how you rate against other people around the world and try to improve your ranking. Or take part in a rowing marathon. For more on indoor competition against yourself or others look at IDEA 28, *Try a Tri.*

Try another idea...

Not strictly speaking a training strategy, but don't forget Sir Steve Redgrave's famous words on winning at the 1996 Atlanta Olympics: 'If anyone sees me anywhere near a boat, they have permission to shoot me.' Of course he went on to win again in 2000 (seemingly without anyone taking a pot shot at him). Never give up on the rower, just look for a new challenge to brighten the routine.

Defining idea...

Q **It's too hard!**

A *Try an easier variation. Don't be ashamed to start your pyramid with one minute bursts and work from there if it makes you more likely to complete the set.*

Q **I'm working flat out but not getting better. How can I make that next step up?**

A *Either you're expecting results too fast, or your problem may be style rather than strength. Go back to IDEA 7 and check the style notes and mistakes in the How did it go? section. Then try stroke golf (above).*

Q **How come my ranking isn't improving against the others?**

A *Maybe they're improving too. If you think about it this can only mean that you're all winning.*

9

Run like Radcliffe I: Fartlek

Stop sniggering. This is how to make the treadmill seem less of a, well, treadmill. If you're already a gym regular you won't need to be told that aside from injury the biggest threat to success is boredom. Walkmans and TV screens may help distract you but they're there because cardiovascular work like cycling on an exercise bike or plugging away on the rowing machine can soon become mind-numbingly dull.

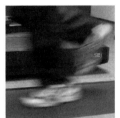

Worst of all has to be running on the treadmill — a term which is in itself a byword for tedious and grinding routine.

That's partly because it's so easy to fall into the common trap of thinking that treadmill running is about one of two things: either running faster, or running for longer. Running faster certainly ups the heartbeat and gets the lungs working but it's intimidating for newcomers, hard to keep up for long, and eventually hits a ceiling as you find your top speed (or in some gyms the speed limit of the machine itself). Running for longer is great for stamina, burning calories (running is one of the most efficient calorie-burning exercises in the gym), and developing those slow-twitch muscle fibres. Which would be great but for the fact that on a treadmill there isn't so much as the slightest shift in the scenery to relieve the tedium of endlessly legging it like a particularly large upright hamster.

TVs in gyms are ideal for fartlek. Try to run at above race pace for the duration of the next music video, or keep running at an incline until the next male vocalist takes to the screen. If it's sport on screen, then set your treadmill speed up a notch for each successful pass completed or, if you're particularly masochistic, try keeping up your race pace until your own team slots it into the back of the net.

Which is where fartlek comes in. All right, all right, settle down at the back there. Yes, it may sound silly but in fact it's Swedish for *speedplay* (rather than something you'd find in the Ikea catalogue). The technique is credited to a Swedish running coach, Gosta Holmer, who was responsible for producing a swathe of speedy Scandinavians who promptly walked (very quickly) all over the competition in the 1950s. The idea couldn't be simpler – more varied, more interesting and more challenging running results in better runners.

Most of us, left to our own devices, tend to do the same kind of run over and over. That becomes particularly clear in the gym where the majority of treadmill sessions involve dialling in a speed and plodding away until the assigned time is up. Which is OK up to a point, but ultimately only trains you to do that exact same run, at that exact same level of effort.

The idea of fartlek is to vary pace and effort, rewarding bursts of extra hard work with recovery periods at an easier rate. That's the speed part of speedplay. The play part comes in by throwing in an element of unpredictability. Fartlek runners in the open air may decide to sprint to a lamppost and then take it easy to the next one as a means of varying the effort. To add to the fun, fartlekers might decide to run faster as soon as they pass, say, a man with a dog, and not slow down until they pass the next baby-buggy. As a result fartlek sessions are not measured in distance covered or speed but in the time of the session.

FARTLEKING AROUND

In the gym there aren't usually a lot of baby-buggies or men with dogs, but what you do have is a treadmill capable of different speeds and angles of climb. Instead of your normal run, try warming up gently for five to ten minutes then increasing the gradient dramatically for five minutes, or sprinting the next half a kilometre at a speed a good couple of notches up from your usual. As for the element of the unexpected, you usually have a whole gym-full of suspects who can unwittingly be roped in. You've probably upped the tempo at some time because you got a bit competitive with the person running on the machine next to you. Or there was someone passing by who you wanted to impress. Well it may be childish, but it's not necessarily bad technique. Try setting a goal like sprinting for as long as the huge guy in the corner can manage to bench press those car-sized weights. Or give yourself a rest period jogging gently for as long as that lycra-sheathed individual takes to get a drink at the fountain.

Whatever it takes. A good session should include a mix of alternated easy running, hard running, hill climbing, walking and absolutely flat out. What you should resist is the temptation to jog along idly, sprint for a minute at the end, and declare that you've just completed a half-hour fartlek session. How much you get out depends very much on how much you put in.

Try another idea...

Looking for more ways to brighten up treadmill time? Then take a look at IDEA 10, *Run like Radcliffe II*, to learn about how intervals can help you predict that marathon you've been daydreaming of.

Defining idea...

'Mixing the pace of your runs can add a whole new dimension to your training. Try increasing the pace of your running between two landmarks as you run; this allows your body to become accustomed to running at a variety of paces.'
PAULA RADCLIFFE

Aside from the light relief of varying your routines (and never underestimate the importance of that), the great benefit of fartlek is that it prepares you for the unexpected. Some time you're not going to be on a treadmill, you're going to be out there in the real world where there are barking dogs to accelerate away from, attractive members of the opposite sex to impress and wildly unpredictable running partners to keep up with. Should you ever want to take part in a race you'll find that having a variety of paces helps enormously in dealing with the human bottleneck at the start or the need to outpace a challenging runner who's making a move to overtake you. Just remember that when talking to non-runners it's better to call it 'speedplay', not 'fartlek', unless of course you're comfortable about having your would-be admirers collapse into a fit of snorting giggles.

How did it go?

Q   I've tried fartlek and it seems a lot like interval training. Is it the same?

A   *If it seems similar, then you're not doing enough to make it unpredictable. The key difference between fartlek and interval training is the random element of letting outside factors decide how fast and far you run.*

Q   I've included short sprints with the gradient set to maximum but I'm getting a sore foot. Am I doing something wrong?

A   *Normally the softer (compared to the road) surface of a treadmill helps avoid impact injuries but if you're not used to running uphill, then the impact of the ball of your foot on the treadmill can cause sesamoiditis – a pain in the big knobbly bone behind the big toe. It's a trauma injury so the answer is to treat it to an ice pack and take it easy. Try building up more gently in future*

Q   **I've tried this fartlek malarkey and it may be fun but it leaves me a bit sore in my legs. How can I avoid this?**

A   *Are you sure you're warming up adequately? Because of the sudden changes in effort level and the fact that you're deliberately surprising your muscles, it's all the more important to warm up thoroughly and start off each session with a gentle jog to get you going.*

Q   **I've tried this fartlek thing and I barely break a sweat. Is that right?**

A   *While no one said it has to hurt, and there's always a time and place for gentle workouts, you'll get the most benefit by mixing and matching 'rest' modes with bursts of hard work that may well exceed your usual levels of effort.*

Q   **I find running uphill on the machine really hard work. Is it worth it?**

A   *In a word, yes. Many professional runners set a slight incline anyway when running on treadmills to compensate for the lack of wind resistance. By getting your muscles and joints used to varying conditions you can strengthen them so that you are less likely to injure yourself when faced with unexpected uphills in the great outdoors.*

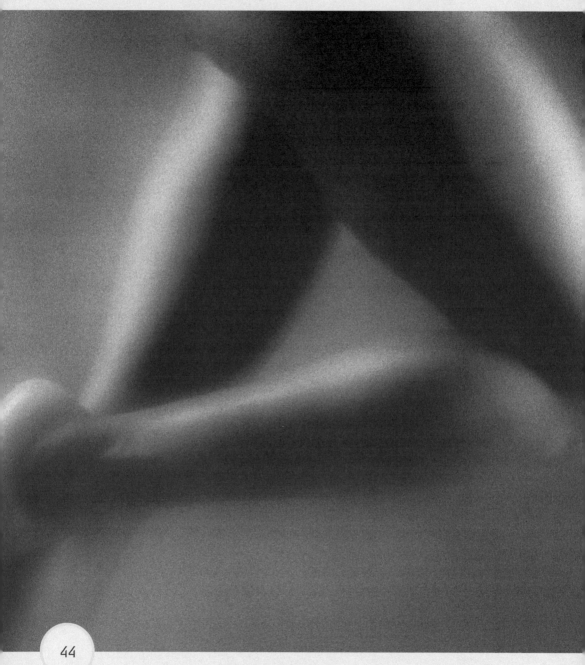

10
Run like Radcliffe II: Yasso 800s

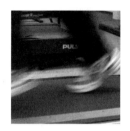

Never done a marathon and curious if you could hit that time you hanker after? Looking to improve your existing marathon times? Well here's how to know if you can do either – without having to run the legendary 42.4 km (26.2 miles).

The idea of interval training revolves around the fact that there's more to running than just pegging it at the same pace all the time.

By running at above normal pace for short intervals, then resting by running more slowly ('active recovery' as it's known in the trade) you can train yourself to run faster, for longer. Interval training for runners usually seems to involve a track, someone with a stopwatch and a complicated formula of distances and times. Yasso 800s, on the other hand, give you the performance goals of intervals, with a pretty fair idea of whether you could achieve your marathon goal. Best of all, anyone can remember the formula and you can forget about the mental maths and instead concentrate on the running.

Here's an idea for you...

Never seriously thought of running a marathon but can run four or five kilometres? Well go and try a couple of Yasso 800s, see what you can do, and start dreaming about whether you could go for the big one.

Yasso 800s get their name from Bart Yasso, who worked on the US magazine *Runner's World*. During Bart's fifteen years of running marathons he noticed a direct link between his times and the time he took to run a series of 800 m (about half a mile). The idea is simple. Say you've always felt that you had it in you to complete a marathon in the highly respectable time of four hours. Take that goal of four hours and now you have your 800 m goal – only in minutes. Now go to our friend the treadmill and (after warming up) bang out 800 m in four minutes, then 'rest' by dropping the speed and running gently for exactly the same number of minutes. Then you try to do another 800 m in four minutes, then rest for the same time. Bart Yasso starts his Yasso 800s a couple of months before the marathon in question, and starts with a workout of four 800 m sprints and rest periods. He then works it up by adding an extra 800 m sprint to the set until he gets up to ten 800 m sprints with ten rests of the same length. Once he hits that he is confident of being able to achieve his marathon goal.

With Bart Yasso that goal is somewhere around 2 hours 40 minutes but the odd thing is that the same principle seems to work whatever your speed. If you think it would take five hours to go the distance, then working on five minute 800s should see you through. If your heart is set on 3 hours 27 minutes then your 800s should be rolling off in 3 minutes 27 seconds. Admit it, once you've set your goal you're not going to have trouble remembering what time you're meant to run 800 m intervals in. Just one thing to remember though. Bart Yasso runs his 800 m on a outdoors track, you are running yours on a treadmill with no wind resistance. To compensate for that you should up the treadmill incline to 1 per cent.

The Yasso can also be a reality check to help rein in the overambitious. For example, if you're thinking of running a sub-three-hour marathon, then you should be aware that to do the Yasso 800s you will need to run those 800 m sets at a treadmill speed of just over 16 kilometres per hour – which is ten miles an hour or six-minute miling.

If you want to know a little more about interval training and what it can do for you then try IDEA 37, *The cardio cocktail*.

Try another idea...

Of course this is running, not rocket science, and critics have attacked the simplicity of the approach, claiming that it doesn't take into account VO2 max, lactate thresholds or cruise intervals. What these critics don't get, or don't like, is that most of us don't understand or wish to understand what VO2 max or lactate thresholds are. We just want to know whether we have a cat's chance of reaching that elusive marathon goal.

The long and the short is that the Yasso technique isn't guaranteed to be 100 per cent accurate because (a) we're all made differently (thank heavens) and as (b) one person's idea of resting running between sprints is another person's idea of sprinting. Yasso 800s may get one person to their target time within fractions of a second and another runner may find

'I've been doing this particular workout for about 15 years and it always seems to work for me. If I can get my 800s down to two minutes 50 seconds, I'm in 2:50 marathon shape.'
BURT YASSO

Defining idea...

themselves a few minutes out. But enough quibbling, it's a proven favourite, it's accurate enough for all but the hardcore and even I can remember what it involves. Which is a noted improvement on previous attempts at interval training which involved having to keep a manual to hand.

How did it go?

Q **The treadmill in my gym takes forever to slow down and speed up. How can I break the run up into neat three/four/five minute segments?**

A *Are you trying to slow down hugely from your race speed? If you need to drop to a much lower rest speed, then you may be overstretching yourself.*

Q **I can't run the *first* 800 m in my target time, let alone ten. What am I doing wrong?**

A *Maybe you're going to have to accept that your target time is a little over-optimistic. Not being able to run ten at once is normal, but if you fancy yourself for a four-hour marathon and can't run a four-minute 800 m, then you may have to readjust your targets.*

Q **How come I can run four 800 m but the fifth is impossible?**

A *Are you sure you're ready to add the fifth? You shouldn't add any more 800 m sprints to the set until you are clearly completing the previous sprint within the target time. Human nature makes it tempting to gloss over those few seconds here or there and impatiently add another set before we're ready. If a new set is suddenly way too hard, then keep on with the previous number and concentrate on doing them easily before adding another.*

Q **I'm running a marathon in six months' time. Should I start my Yasso's now?**

A *It's fine to try a few 800 m sessions to get a feel for your goals, but strictly speaking the Yasso approach is aimed at fine-tuning closer to the race and after having put in the distance work.*

11

Balls I: Great balls of rubber

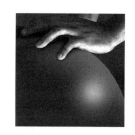

Ever wondered what those oversized beach ball things are doing in the gym? Well here's where you find out what they're for, and why a bit of ball-play can help create a better you.

Swiss balls are just wonderful. They're big, they're soft, they're squidgy, they come in rainbow colours and they smell great.

Only you're going to have to take my word on what they smell like because they're so obviously meant to appeal to kids that you probably haven't dared use one yet. Well here's the good news: you can get comfy, play ball and roll around on the floor with confidence because those balls are the key to great stretches and core strength. Which translates to a flat stomach – something that at least half the people in any gym are working towards, only they don't know how to use the balls.

The first thing to know about the balls is that they aren't all the same size. Different balls are suitable for different sized people. The key is being able to sit comfortably on top of the ball with your knees bent and your feet flat on the floor. Roughly speaking a 45 cm diameter ball suits people 1.40–1.52 m tall (4 feet 7 inches–5 feet in old money); 55 cm balls are for those 1.55–1.68 m tall (5 feet 1 inch–5 feet 6 inches),

Here's an idea for you... **If you find the side stretch comfortable, then at the top of the stretch, when you are resting on your side, try twisting your torso to turn face down onto the ball so that your chest and both arms are resting on it.**

and 65 cm for people who are 1.70–1.80 m tall (5 feet 7 inches to 5 feet 11 inches). There are 75 cm balls for the six-footers (1.83 m) and even an 85 cm ball for basketballers but you will probably have to buy one from the US. Generally the balls you see in gyms are 65 cm with a few smaller ones around. Manufacturers colour code their balls by size, but beware: your gym may have bought from different manufacturers so that nice small yellow ball that was just right may turn out to be oddly larger next time you reach for it. Two important things to know about the ball. One: they are tougher than you think and can take a full-grown man and all the weight he can heft on a pair of dumbbells. Two: although you can burst them if you press them onto something sharp they don't explode, but just deflate pathetically, so don't be afraid to bounce on them.

Swiss balls are soft and supportive, as you will feel as you lay yourself out across one, which means you can trust yourself to one and stretch in comfort. Balls being balls, however, are round and so everything you do perched on the ball involves a little bit of balancing, and this means working the muscles that control your core stability, even if all you're doing is sitting on the thing.

EXERCISES TO TRY

You may be tempted just to sit on the ball while watching telly, but there are more effective ways to exercise to develop stretches, core stability and strength (for which see IDEA 12, *Balls II*).

SIDE STRETCH

Kneel with the ball next to you and your arm resting on it. Now with the leg that's furthest from the ball stretch straight out sideways and gently shift the weight onto the ball so you are draped over it sideways on. The hand that's not on the ball should now stretch up and over your head towards the ball.

Enjoy using the ball for stretching? Now try it for strength work in IDEA 12, *Balls II*.

Try another idea...

BACK STRETCH

Sit on the centre of the ball, making sure that your feet are a little apart to keep you rock solid and stable. Then very gently walk your feet away so that you lie back and both your back and neck come down to be supported on the ball. You may want to have a hand behind your head to take the weight off your neck until it is resting on the ball. With your feet flat on the floor, now open your arms on each side and feel the stretch across your back. To open it up a bit more, stretch your arms over your head and down as if reaching for the floor behind your head.

FORWARD ROLL OUT

Kneel on the floor in front of your ball and lean forward very slightly to rest your forearms on the ball with your hands together. Now, keeping the abs good 'n' tight, gently roll the ball forward until your arms are straight. Hold that for a moment, then roll it back to the start position. Repeat. Most people find that although the body position is very comfortable, the exercise is surprisingly hard on their stomach muscles.

'Happiness is a ball after which we run wherever it rolls, and we push it with our feet when it stops.'
JOHANN WOLFGANG VON GOETHE

Defining idea...

51

How did it go?

Q **I tried the back stretch and it feels great once in position. But why does my neck hurt as I lie back to start the stretch?**

A *If your neck hurts, then support the weight of your head with your hands as you lie back.*

Q **I like the forward roll out, but don't find it challenging enough for my abs. How can I up the ante?**

A *If you want to make it more difficult, and you have a strong back, then you can try going up onto the points of your feet instead of your knees.*

Q **I'm told just sitting on the ball is beneficial. Can that be true?**

A *Yes, sitting on the ball involves lots of small balancing moves (or big ones if you lift your feet of the floor) so in theory even watching the telly while balanced on the ball will work your core stability.*

12
Balls II:
The balls bounce back

In IDEA 11, *Balls I*, you saw how those oversized beach balls can actually help with your stretching. Here you find out that they can also be used for strength work. So forget the fun and games, this is where the balls get their own back.

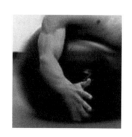

Flip through the glossy pages of the exercise magazines and sooner or later you'll see a picture of a muscle man or lycra lady sitting happily on a Swiss ball working a dumbbell in each hand.

This is both good and bad. The good is that while it may look as if they are just using the ball as a convenient object for a quick sit-down, the theory behind this practice is sound. Dumbbell workouts such as biceps curls or flies for the shoulders and chest will benefit from being done on the ball, though not perhaps where you expect. Even though the ball is dead comfy to sit on it is nonetheless inherently unstable. Which means that as you exercise on it you are making minute adjustments all the time in order to keep your balance. With weights in your hands those adjustments are exaggerated, and so your midsection, and in particular the deep-lying stomach muscles, are getting a workout as you work the arms. Two for the price of one. One tip though – since the whole benefit is dependent on being

Here's an idea for you...

Got the hang of this balancing thing? Finding it all too easy? Then try a wall-hanging reverse crunch, to work those lower abs a bit harder. You'll need to move the ball to a position near the wall bars so you can lie across the ball with your lower back on it while your hands stretch out above your head to grip the wall bars. Your legs should be bent with your feet on the floor. Now lift your knees up into your chest as you would with a normal reverse crunch. You'll not only have to lift them but also balance them (did I mention that you're lying on top of a ball?).

slightly off balance you should always try to work the arms asymmetrically. So, for example, when performing biceps curls the left arm should be bending as the right straightens.

There is, however, just one catch in the real world when it comes to performing biceps curls on the ball. Where are you going to get those dumbbells from?

It's true that some gyms, particularly those with a separate ladies section, will have a selection of small fixed-weight dumbbells near to the stretching mats where the Swiss balls live. That doesn't help the blokes much though, and for most gyms there is a strict system of apartheid in place whereby the dumbbells live in the free weights room (all grunting men with muscles) while the Swiss balls live by the stretching area (lots more lycra and elegance). Try taking the dumbbells off their racks and walking away and someone will (with some reason) protest. Try walking into the free weights room, that sanctuary of testosterone and steroids, with a brightly coloured, oversize beach ball and you might just as well announce that you'll take on everyone in the room. However much we'd all like to see someone break that particular rule the chances are that unless you have the confidence, or the physique of a 200-kilo gorilla, you will never break the never-the-twain-shall-meet rule of the weights and stretching equipment.

Which leaves you with just one option for strength training on the ball. Using yourself as a weight. The following are all variations on tried and trusted strength moves, only with the subtle addition of a large vinyl ball. See if you can spot the difference.

Finding it difficult to build up to large numbers of repetitions? You may want to try a routine that works on light weights lifted often, such as BodyPump – see IDEA 33, Pump that body.

Try another idea...

THE PUSH-UP

Standard push-ups are the mainstay of the workout routine for everybody from the army to the long-term inmate. This one takes that exercise into a different dimension, oh and no hard core convict would be seen dead with a bouncy ball as a training partner.

Simply adopt the standard face-down press-up position, only with your knees on the ball (or your ankles if you're a press-up powerhouse). Now bend your elbows and lower your face towards the floor and straighten to get back up – all slowly and with control. Repeat as often as you would a normal press-up but notice where you can feel the squeeze.

'Perform your work with minimum effort and maximum pleasure.'
JOSEPH H. PILATES

Defining idea...

By raising the feet above the level of the floor you put more of your bodyweight onto your arms, which works the triceps, and the tilt throws the effort more onto the upper part of the chest. We're not finished there though. Because your feet aren't only raised, but balancing on a ball, you'll also have to correct the wobbles, meaning that you will tense and work your abdominals as you go.

THE JACK-KNIFE

This looks like a distorted press-up but if you think about it it's really just a reverse crunch (where you bring your knees up to your chest) only turned upside down. Assume the press-up position, again with your feet together on the ball, only this time keep your arms straight and bend your knees, gently rolling the ball towards you. Now straighten out your legs to get you and the ball back to where they were. Control is the key here and you should quickly feel that most of the effort is coming from your midsection.

You want more? Easy, just combine them – one press-up, then without changing position perform the jack-knife, then the press-up again.

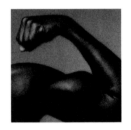

Q   **I've tried the ball but don't feel at all confident with the lack of balance. What can I do to get over this?**

A   *Practice makes perfect, but if you're feeling wobbly then don't try to do the strength exercises just yet. Go back to Balls I and concentrate on feeling at ease with stretching on the ball before you try to add strength work to the mix.*

Q   **I've pretty much got the hang of press-ups on the ball but can only do about five or six before collapsing with the effort. How do I work on doing more?**

A   *The further down your legs the ball is, the harder the effort. If you currently rest your shins on the ball, then try moving it forward towards your knees (or even your thighs if necessary) until you can do ten or more repetitions. Then gently move the ball further back as your arms, shoulders and chest get stronger.*

Q   **My gym has several sizes of Swiss ball and I have been told to use the smaller one, does this apply to the press-up as well?**

A   *In a word, no. The correct 'size' of Swiss ball per person is related to your height and how you sit on it (see IDEA 11, Balls I). Here you aren't sitting on it and the only difference the size makes is that a larger ball tips more of the weight onto your shoulders and upper chest than a smaller ball would do.*

How did
it go?

57

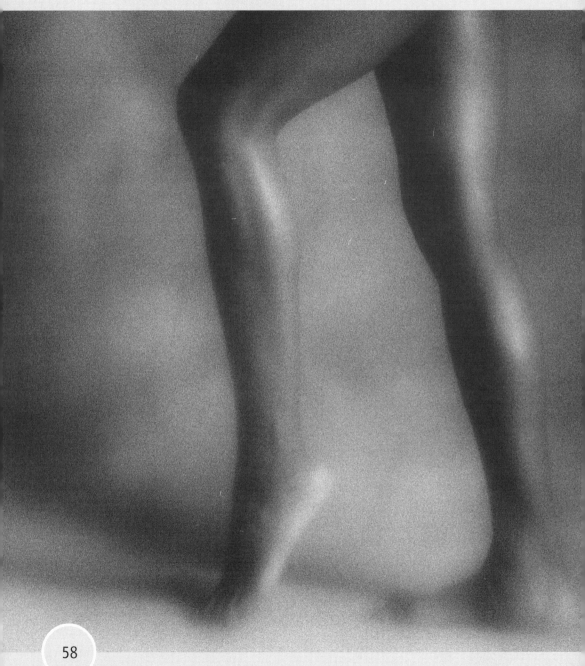

13

Stairway to heaven

Everyone knows that the stepper is how you forge buns of steel, but a select few also know how to get a full fat-burning cardio and core-strength workout at the same time. Shhh...here's the secret.

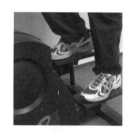

However fit I think I am, a run up steps leaves me gasping for air like a stranded fish.

Unless I'm indeed unique (and I don't think I am) there are a lot of us who are reminded every day of what a dramatic workout something as simple as a flight of stairs can provide. Yet when it's office chucking-out time and the gyms are suddenly chocka there is pretty much always a free stepper sulking in a corner somewhere. The humble stepper is possibly the most underused and ill-used piece of kit in the whole gym, and all because of a simple misunderstanding about how to use it.

To come at the stepper from a different angle (from behind to be precise), let's consider what exactly it is working. While steppers differ slightly from each other in design and the way they provide resistance, the bottom (sorry) line is that they present you with resistance which you overcome by pressing down or stepping up with alternate legs. To do that your body has to recruit a number of muscles, most notably the gluteus maximus, medius and minimus, known collectively to gym bunnies as the *glutes*, and to everyone else as your bum. Because of this most people see the stepper as a means of toning the buttocks, and for some reason that means that it is largely left to the women. This is presumably some kind of throwback to the

Here's an idea for you...

Most people looking to push themselves simply up the resistance, but here's another approach. With the resistance fairly low, try upping the ante on yourself by pumping the steps faster, running or pedalling on the spot. Imagine a world in which, for some reason known only unto the French, Tour de France riders compete on unicycles and you are now sprinting against Lance Armstrong for the title of King of the Mountains. Now watch those calories burn off.

days when men honestly believed that biceps were what attracted the opposite sex.

Which leaves us with a couple of people desultorily bobbing up and down on the stepper while a couple of doors down there are rooms full of men and women doing traditional leg exercises such as lunges and squats or queuing for half an hour to get on the treadmill.

Let them. Because the fewer people who understand the potential of the stepper, the more machines there are for the rest of us.

The first thing to understand is that stairs are hard work because we are supporting our own bodyweight and lifting it up, making each step a mini-lunge or squat. Up the resistance of the stepper so you have to launch yourself a little harder and you now have a tough workout for the quads at the front of your thighs and the calves at the back of your legs. Upping the resistance also takes the stepper into serious cardio workout territory – which shouldn't come as a surprise to those of us who get out of breath going upstairs. Last, but not at all least, comes the biggest single tip of standout stepping. It's breathtakingly simple, very little known (judging by the gyms I go to) and changes absolutely everything. You ready for this? OK, here it comes. *Just. Let. Go.*

Give it some and let go, that's all there is to it. You see people hanging off steppers in all sorts of ways, resting their bodyweight on their arms (bad for the wrists), or hanging off backwards. What you don't see are people who let go and use their arms as counterbalances to their pumping legs.

Let go, and now your legs are taking all your bodyweight which massively increases the strength and cardio benefits. Letting go forces you to balance which brings in all the muscles of the torso – obliques, abs and back – and builds up core strength. No matter how quickly or slowly you go you'll now burn far more calories in a much shorter period of time. With all your weight on your legs (and thus driving the stepper) you will burn calories at around twice the rate you get on a stationary bike and not so much less than when you're on the treadmill. Unlike the treadmill, however, the stepper remains a very low-impact activity with minimal shock on the joints. Even serious runners can benefit from the stepper as a way of upping the 'mileage' in their leg muscles without overloading knees or provoking shin splints.

Looking to burn fat without the impact of running on the treadmill? Try bringing in your upper body as well for an all over tone up by giving the elliptical trainer a go (see IDEA 18, *Total ellipse*).

Try another idea...

'The journey of a thousand miles starts with a single step.'
MAO TSE TUNG, the Great Leader, no stranger to lycra hotpants and sweaty towels.

Defining idea...

61

How did it go?

Q   I let go but wobbled all over the shop and nearly fell off. How do I stay on?

A   *Try letting go progressively. Just leave one hand lightly resting in front of you on the bar. When you've cracked that, then work towards keeping just a fingertip balancing you on the machine, and then before you know it it'll be 'look ma, no hands'.*

Q   Without the bar to grip I'm finding it hard to push down against the steps. What am I doing wrong?

A   *If you needed to grip the machine to push down, then you are probably using a very high level of resistance. While this is effective for strength training you may want to try lowering the resistance and upping your speed to get more cardio benefit.*

Q   I've got the hang of this letting go thing and am ploughing happily on. Now what?

A   *As our muscles adapt to an exercise and get better at it they become more efficient and use fewer calories. So keep yourself on your toes by chopping and changing. Most steppers have a random setting which increases or lowers the resistance. Set the machine to 'random' and then cover up the display with a towel so you don't see the changes coming.*

14

Static crackle

Sit-ups, crunches, reverse crunches – have you ever wondered if there was another way to a strong mid-section without all the bobbing up and down? Well there is, and oddly enough it involves not moving at all. Time to get static.

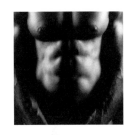

Whether it's about body building or fitness training, the emphasis down the gym tends to be on moving things. Moving heavy things very slowly.

Moving light things very fast. Or simply moving yourself as fast or slowly as you are able. What tends to be forgotten in all this is the potential strength benefits of not moving at all. Welcome to the wonderful world of isometric exercise.

Most exercises are dynamic, and consist of a force moving an object whether that is a weight, some kind of resistance device or just hauling our own sorry selves around. That makes perfect sense because we are moving beasties and good exercise mimics the tasks we have to do in daily life. Or at least the ones we used to do when daily life involved running after mammoths, fleeing things with big pointy teeth and so on. But movement isn't the only way to build muscle, and that's where isometric exercises come in.

Here's an idea for you...

Enjoy the side plank but find it too easy? OK, then to put a bit of a stretch down the other side of the body assume the position and stick your 'spare' arm straight out sideways so it points at the ceiling. Now stretch the arm further over your head so you look something like a sugar plum fairy ballerina who has fallen over sideways in mid pirouette and is too shocked to get up. Hold the position for as long as you can.

Isometrics really mean tensing a muscle without moving anything – either just by contracting it, or by applying a force to something that simply can't go anywhere. Stand in a doorway and try to push the frame apart Samson style. Nothing is moving (hopefully) but, my, can you feel the squeeze. Because it is seen as better to exercise a muscle through its full range of movement, isometric exercises aren't usually recommended for fitness fans unless they've suffered injury to a joint and want to maintain strength. There is, however, one exception. The plank. With the plank and its sideways-on variants the whole point is to hold the body perfectly still. Because it's only supported on the ground at a couple of points, however, this requires quite a lot of muscular effort. Unlike crunches, which mainly work the rectus abdominis, the effort of keeping the stomach straight (and off the ground) requires the work of all the muscles including the obliques and the transversus abdominis. Which makes for a strong midsection.

Purists argue that this isn't really isometric exercise because the muscles are resisting something that can move – as you find out when you stop resisting and collapse like a burst balloon – but who has time for nit-picking when there's gym-fun to be had?

THE PLANK

Couldn't be simpler. Lie face down on a mat and then lift up so you are resting your weight on your forearms and your toes (or your knees if toes proves too hard). Now hold that position absolutely rigidly. Your back should be straight – if your bum is sticking up, pull it back into line. If your hips or belly are sagging, then whip them back into line too. You are straight as a ramrod, and by now probably starting to feel about as stiff. Keep going for as long as you can – time yourself and see if you can get any better.

THE SIDE PLANK

This time you start on your side and raise yourself onto your elbow with your body dead straight so that there is a long wedge of daylight underneath you from your elbow (which should be directly under your shoulder) right down to your feet. This puts more of the stress on the sides (surprise) and thus the obliques. If you want to add a bit of extra interest (go on, you know you want to) then stretch the arm that's away from the floor up straight out sideways so its sticks up in the air. When you can't hold it anymore roll over to your other side and repeat the process.

Enjoying developing abs and core strength? OK, maybe enjoying isn't the right word, but if at least you see the importance and can't bear any more crunching, then take a look at the IDEAS 11 and 12, *Balls I* and *Balls II*, as well as IDEA 19, *Roman revenge*.

Try another idea...

'Mastering others is strength. Mastering yourself is true power.'
LAO TZU

Defining idea...

65

How did
it go?

Q **I can hold the position for about ten seconds. Is this any good?**

A *In a word, no. If the full plank is too hard, then try putting your weight on your knees instead of your feet and building up strength by maintaining that position for as long as possible. When you get up to a half minute or so, try going for the full plank.*

Q **My back hurts as I do the plank ...**

A *OK, stop right there. If your back muscles hurt as you try to hold the position, then you must work on strengthening them first. It's even possible that your stomach muscles are too strong for your back and causing an imbalance. Start with IDEA 15, Good morning Superman.*

Q **Does the plank completely replace all those crunches?**

A *No it doesn't, but it works the stomach muscles in a different way from crunching so not only can it help them develop but it'll add a bit of variety to your training diet. Isometric exercises are really a bonus, they don't replace exercises that take muscles through their full natural range of movement.*

15

Good morning superman

Working hard for a flat stomach but neglecting your back muscles? Well neglect your back and no one will see your six-pack or admire your navel piercing because you'll be hunched up like Quasimodo doing his shoelaces.

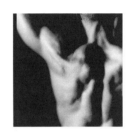

It's one of the simplest but smartest features of our body that most muscles have an opposite muscle that's just as important. Where one pulls, the other pushes.

Your biceps bend your arm, your triceps straighten it out. Most exercises are designed to work both, either in tandem, or one after the other, so as not to create an imbalance. In one key area, however, that rule seems to go out of the window. In the quest for the hard body we tend to spend a lot of time worrying about rock-hard bellies, but forget that unless we strengthen the spinal muscles to cope we could be sowing the seeds of serious back trouble. It's a tribute to the awesome power of vanity really – we all know what a six-pack is, but when was the last time you saw someone on *Baywatch* with just, like, awesome erector spinae? The first most of us know about our back muscles is when they fail on us. Building up the stomach muscles can actually help provoke that by adding to the imbalance between the muscles that curl up the back and the muscles that straighten it. So even if they're not going to win you admiring glances from the opposite sex it pays to put a bit of effort into your back.

Here's an idea for you... **Try doing the Superman-style back extension on a Swiss ball (see IDEA 11, *Balls I*). With your feet firmly on the floor (well, as firmly as you're going to get balanced on a ball) lie face down on the ball so it supports your stomach and ribs. Now lift your head and shoulders off the ball and curve your back upwards. As a variation you can try this with either your hands on your head, or to make it slightly harder, stretch your arms out ahead of you. For a little more effort you can hold light dumbbells in your hands.**

PUTTING YOUR BACK INTO IT

When people talk about the back muscles they usually mean the ones that show towards the tops of the shoulders. Men in particular are fond of working the lats (laterals) that help give a V-shaped torso. The muscles that get ignored, however, are the erector spinae which run up the length of the spine and help hold up upright and straighten the back. It's your erector spinae you reach for when you feel something go in your back. For most of us it's only at that moment that we even think of exercising our back muscles. Which is part of the phenomena that sees some four out of five adults suffering from lower back pain. The more you're working the rest of your body, the more you need a strong back to hold it all together.

Just one thing though. Kill or cure is not the way to work in a gym, so before working your back you should be sure to have sought out qualified medical advice and talked it over with the gym instructors. You have? Promise? OK, over to you.

SUPERMAN – OR INDEED SUPERWOMAN

Lie flat on your front on a mat and smoothly lift both your arms and your feet off the mat as if you were trying to curl your whole body into a bow shape with only your stomach, ribs and hips left on the mat. Keep it steady, hold it for a moment, then return. Now add a slight twist to that by slowly raising your right arm with your left leg, then your left arm with your right leg. This should be comfortable enough to do ten or twenty times without feeling difficulty.

GOOD MORNING

The name of this exercise suggests that it goes back to a particularly courteous bygone age since really what you are about to do is take a bow. Stand with your feet shoulder-width apart and your knees slightly bent. Bend forward from the waist until your torso is parallel to the floor and hold this position for a moment before gently rising back up. If you feel great doing this, then you can add weight to the exercise with either a very light barbell across your shoulders or a light dumbbell in each hand with the weight resting on each shoulder. If you are a beginner to back workouts or feel anything that could remotely be described as a twinge, then don't even think about the weights.

If you're a glutton for punishment you can go to the Roman Chair (see IDEA 19, *Roman revenge*) and instead of lying on your back to work your abs you can flip over on to your front and work on extending and contracting your back. Don't even think about doing this unless your back is already strong, and remember that you've already promised to take qualified medical advice before working your back.

Try another idea...

'*You are as young as the flexibility of your spine.*'
JOSEPH H. PILATES

Defining idea...

69

How did it go?

Q **My back hurts when I do any of these exercises. What should I do now?**

A *Golden rule: if your back hurts, then back off. Remember you promised to take advice before doing these, and if you find that doing Supermans causes you pain, then it's straight off to the osteopath for you.*

Q **Supermans are too easy. Can I make them more challenging?**

A *If you're really confident that your back is strong, then you can move on to doing back exercises with dumbbells in your hands to increase the load. Remember to start small and be very conservative in increasing the load – the idea is to avoid back trouble, not to provoke it.*

Q **Can lower back exercises cause the muscle to bulk up?**

A *No. Some muscles just don't bulk up, otherwise talkative people would have giant tongues. If your body fat percentage is low enough you may be able to see the results but not as bulging muscle, just as a more toned look.*

16
On yer (stationary) bike I: Style

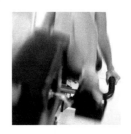

Sitting on a stationary bike flipping through the *Financial Times* isn't going to cut it when it comes to fat-burning or fitness.

Try some triathlon cyclist techniques for getting better instead of just getting bored.

If you've read IDEA 5, *Quality versus quantity*, you'll have come across the idea of junk training. If you really want to see an orgy of junk training in action just go and check out what's happening on the stationary bikes in most gyms. Of course it's possible that every one is a blur of blistering biking, but if your gym is anything like mine there's at least one person reading a book, while a couple of others begrudgingly nudge the pedals with all the enthusiasm of someone who's just given up looking for the 'freewheel' setting. Until the day they invent the stationary tandem you don't have to worry about the quality of anyone else's stationary bike bashing, but if you recognise yourself as one of the above, then it's time to get better, before boredom gets the better of you.

Here's an idea for you... **Once you've got a more efficient stroke right through the cycle, try working one leg at a time. You don't have to take the other foot off the pedal, just be strict about only pushing with one leg. Now try and keep up the revolution count. You'll find that as you get better at working all the way through the stroke you can maintain a higher speed than you did when you used to just push down.**

COUNTER REVOLUTIONARY

The stationary bike has many things going for it – it provides a great low-impact cardio workout – but the features that attract most of us are: (a) you get to sit down; and (b) unlike all those scary looking machines at least you know what you're supposed to do on a stationary bike.

Sitting down is a great position for resting – literally taking the weight off your legs – but taking your bodyweight out of the equation has serious consequences when it comes to calorie burning. Moderate effort on an exercise bike will burn around half the calories of running on a treadmill or giving it hell on a stepper (see IDEA 13, *Stairway to heaven*).

As for point (b), years of riding bicycles mean that we tend to think that as long as the pedals are making little circles, then we're probably doing what we should. And since that doesn't exactly demand 100 per cent attention, we then reach for the nearest copy of *Hello!*

Instead of trying to tune out, try some professional cyclist tips for improving your technique (and in the process powering up your hip flexors and bum muscles.)

FIRST OFF, A QUICK NOTE ON FORM

On the upright bike, make sure you've got the seat adjusted so that your knee is very slightly bent at the bottom of the stroke. A completely straight leg suggests you may have trouble reaching the pedal, and a very bent knee at the bottom of the stroke will put real pressure on your joints.

Next sit upright – don't be tempted to lean forward and rest your weight on your wrists or elbows. Never mind what those whip-thin little pros do on the telly, we don't have any wind resistance to work against here and we're not on enough drugs to blot out the back pain that comes from bad posture.

Make sure those foot-straps are good and tight – you're going to need them.

Got this one cracked – great, now take your silky smooth cycling skills and try some of the resistance work drills in IDEA 17, *On yer bike – II: Strength*.

Try another idea...

THEY'RE OFF! – CYCLE STYLE

'Ride lots.'
EDDIE MERCKX

Defining idea...

Most of us think that pedalling is a downwards push, followed by a few seconds respite as the pedal comes round, before giving it some again. Bad news: the pros like to work the pull up as well as the push down. The idea is to develop a smooth, circular force that evens out the stroke and leads to more efficient cycling. As a bonus it also recruits more muscles (notably the hamstrings) into the stroke and firms up your bum and thighs.

There are four parts (arcs) to the full circle of your pedal cycle:

1. Down – the bit you're already pushing on.

2. Bottom and back – at the bottom of the stroke, the bit where you probably stop pushing. What you should be doing is pulling back at this point. Imagine you've stepped in something nasty and are scraping it off.

3. Up – harder without being 'clipped-on' with cycle shoes, but you can still pull on this arc if you have those foot-straps done up.

4. Top – imagine the curve at this transition point from pulling up to pushing down.

Now break the stroke down and try to spend a couple of minutes just pushing on stroke 1. That should come easily – after all it's what we normally do – so before getting too complacent, try switching to the second part of the stroke and focusing on putting your effort into that. Next go for the third part, and then the fourth. Inevitably the easiest and most powerful part of the stroke to do will be the down-stroke, but with a bit of practice you should be able to feel a smoother all-round rhythm.

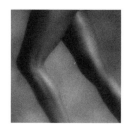

Q **What's the difference between the laid-back and the sit-up-and-beg bikes in the gym, and can I do this drill on both?**

How did it go?

A   *Most gyms feature two types of stationary bike – recumbent (where you're nearly flat on your back), and upright (seated). The principal difference between the recumbent and the upright is that the recumbent offers a backrest which you may find useful if back trouble is the reason you're in the gym in the first place. Since few of us ride recumbent bikes out on the road, however, these drills are really aimed at the upright versions.*

Q **Feels great, get the point, got that circular action thing going – but how do I know if I'm getting any better?**

A   *Switch the computer readout to r.p.m. and see if you can keep the revolutions up when you're putting your power into arcs 2, 3 and 4. Don't worry about speed (it's not usually accurate on exercise bikes), just focus on revs.*

Q **I can do it, I can do it and I've got that rev counter redlining like Schumacher down the home straight. Now what?**

A   *Now up the resistance and see if you can still turn the pedals when you're just pushing/pulling on arcs 2, 3 and 4.*

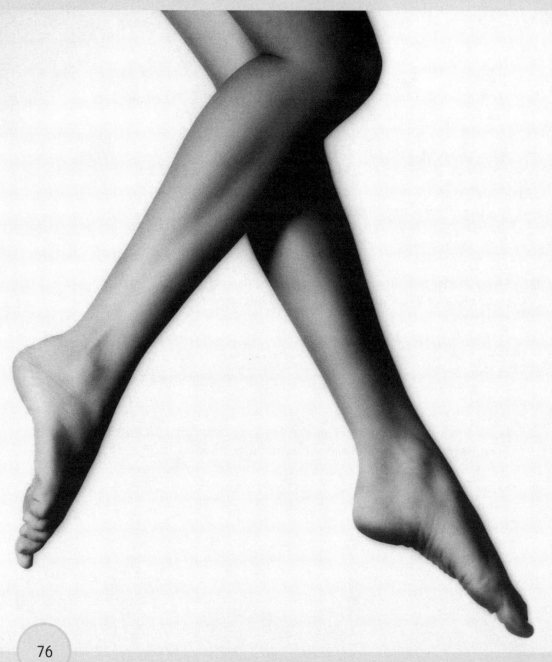

17

On yer (stationary) bike II: Strength

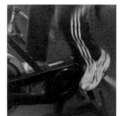

Great, you read Idea 16, *On yer bike I*, and it helped you put down that copy of *Hello!* and work harder than you ever thought possible on a bike that doesn't go anywhere. Now what?

In Idea 16, we looked at style work — making you a better cyclist. Now it's time to turn those skills into raw power by looking at strength work.

There are two key parts to this: *cadence*, which really means how fast you're managing to spin those pedals, and *resistance*, which is how hard the machine is trying to stop you from spinning those pedals. In the quest to become a rounded, multi-skilled, renaissance kind of a gym bunny (and because we get bored easily) we're going to work on both.

CADENCE CADENZA

You've probably heard of spinning classes (and if you haven't take a look at IDEA 45, *In a spin*). In cycling terms 'spinning' is a technique in which you choose a gear that means there is little resistance as you turn it, but you keep the speed up so that you're

Here's an idea for you...

As you get used to short periods of peak effort with this workout, try to combine it with heart monitoring to see how fast your pulse drops back down from its maximum afterwards. Many stationary bikes have built-in heart monitors or you can check your own with the information in IDEA 4, Listen to your love muscle.

spinning the pedals at high speed (100 r.p.m. and more). For long-distance racing cyclists spinning equates to high speeds over a long period, for time-pressed gym users it can mean harder, but more interesting workouts... such as this one:

Start off with a warm-up for five to ten minutes, then make sure you can see the r.p.m./rev readout on the bike's computer. On some models r.p.m./rev may be displayed as part of a rotating selection of information. Make sure you've switched it to r.p.m./rev or 'locked' it on that info because you'll turn the air blue if it flicks over to some other reading just as you're trying to hold an r.p.m. for a fixed time.

Take a good look at what your comfortable cadence is. If it's slower than 90, then try bringing it up to 90 for a couple of minutes to see how that feels.

Now speed up until the rev counter reads 120 (110 if that's too hard) and don't let it drop below that for two minutes.

Drop back to your comfortable cadence for a minute.

Without jerking your feet around or plunging the pedals downwards as if trying to stamp something to death, try accelerating smoothly up to the highest rev reading you can reach. Hold it there for 10–15 seconds, before coming back down equally smoothly to your comfortable cadence.

Out of breath? Good, time to do it all over again. Five times to be exact.

As you get better at this you'll find that you can either reach a higher rev count at the peak, or hold your original high point for longer. Try holding your original max for longer. If you can hold it for 30 seconds to a minute, then it's time to set your sights higher.

RESISTANCE (IS FUTILE?)

Most stationary bikes these days have a whole smorgasbord of settings and odds are one of them will be called something along the lines of 'hill climb'. Hill climb programmes on gym bikes vary, but there's usually a choice between a single long steady up and down and a series of short sharp ups and downs. If you have an option that gives you a series of peaks, then go for that; if not, opt for manual and make your own peaks.

The idea is that the resistance level should leave you feeling comfortable pedalling at the bottom of each 'hill', then working harder as you go up. Right at the top (which should be held for 1–2 minutes) you should feel better if you get up out of the saddle and stand up to pedal. Bingo. Because it's at that stand-up moment that we pull one last little trick on those poor legs. As you stand up to pedal try to 'lock' your whole body absolutely steady so you don't bob up and down at all (it helps if you're opposite a mirror at this point). If your body is rigid and unmoving, then you aren't using your bodyweight to power the down

Like the feel of cadence and resistance? Well then bring them both together in a spinning class – see IDEA 45, *In a spin*.

Try another idea...

'Quite a number of our young men, who formerly were addicted to stupid habits, and seeking of nonsensical distractions and vulgar pleasures, are now vigorous, healthy, energetic, and for the sake of this extraordinary machine submit themselves to an ascetic rule of life, and, induced by taste and passion, acquire habits of temperance, the imperative desire of quiet and regular living, and most important of all, the steady exercise of self-control.'
HENRI DESGRANGES, founder of the Tour de France.

Defining idea...

stroke and, boy, should you feel that in your thigh muscles (quadriceps). Try to hold that position for a minute or two, then drop back down (and lower the resistance if necessary). A series of four or five hills each with a standing 'peak' should give you a workout you'll remember on the way home.

How did
it go?

Q Why can't I get the r.p.m. over 100 now matter how hard I try?

A Fair enough, take it at your own pace and set your goals according to your abilities, but try taking a look at IDEA 16, On yer bike I for techniques and see if you can get more out of each part of your pedalling.

Q I try resistance work and am happy standing on the pedals but can't seem to keep my torso still.

A Concentrate on isolating the movement in the hips. It could be that you have the resistance a little too high so you're recruiting your bodyweight to try and get that extra downward push. Try the hill climbing on a lower setting until you have a smooth technique

Q As I workout I'm also checking on my heart rate – but what sort of intensity should I be working at?

A For resistance and high cadence work you should be in the cardio range of 75-85 per cent of your maximum heart rate – for more on working that out take a look at IDEA 4, Listen to your love muscle.

18

Total ellipse

If you've got a limited amount of time and your goal is fat-burning, or you want a weight-bearing workout that takes in upper and lower body, then the elliptical trainer (sometimes called a cross-trainer) is the baby for you.

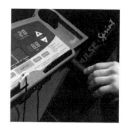

The elliptical trainer is a relatively new kid on the gym block but its popularity means that it's a rare gym without a small posse of them hanging out somewhere near the TV screens.

If you're fighting shy of it because they didn't have them in gyms when you last went, or it looks sort of complicated, then it's high time the two of you got acquainted.

Compared to the other machines in the gym the elliptical trainer has a number of unique advantages. Take a quick look at its neighbours. The rower provides a great upper and lower body workout, but isn't weight bearing, so you don't burn so many calories and you don't build bone density. Then there's the treadmill which is weight bearing at its best, but involves the considerable impact of that weight crashing into the ground with every footfall. The stepper, on the other hand, manages weight-bearing exercise without the impact of running, although it doesn't work your arms. Which only leaves the elliptical as the machine that makes

Although it means forgoing the upper-body benefit of the machine you may want to try jogging on the elliptical. The benefits of this are much as for the *just let go* idea in IDEA 13, *Stairway to heaven* – balance and core strength. The difference is that this movement is much closer to normal running and with even less impact than a stepper. Set the elliptical to a (very) low resistance level and, watching your balance, let go of the handles. Accelerate slowly so as to get used to the elliptical action of the pedals and don't outrun the pedals so your feet lift off (which is why you'll need to be on very low resistance). Now try to 'run' for 2–5 minutes before resuming your normal routine.

you work with your own bodyweight, but no impact (your feet never lift off from the pedals) and using your arms. The result is a high calorie burn rate, and an overall workout that makes it a great warm-up for other exercises.

A FEW TIPS ON FORM

Ellipticals are low impact and the ellipse action makes it hard for you to injure yourself using them but we humans are a remarkably inventive species when it comes to damaging ourselves with inanimate objects. Try to keep your knees slightly bent at all times, they should never lock. Keep your arms relaxed and try not to bounce your body – however much fun you're having.

A FEW TIPS ON FUN

This is a largely self-explanatory machine, with a few variations from one model to another in terms of the programme options on offer. Pretty much all the machines you'll come across have a resistance setting (usually from 1 to 20) and the higher you set that the more work you'll have to do to keep going. In particular on the higher settings you'll have to work harder with your arms to maintain momentum and the twisting effect that has will also give your abs and obliques something of a workout. Try different settings to add a bit of variety to your routine, and notice that the higher the resistance, the higher the number of calories you'll burn to overcome it.

Remember that you have two possible actions with your arms – you can either put your energy into pushing each handle away from you, or into pulling towards you. Pushing will exercise your chest (pectoral) muscles and the backs of your arms (triceps), pulling will put more emphasis on your back (lattisimus dorsi or *lats*) and your biceps. Try mixing and matching with five minutes just pushing, then five minutes just pulling for a more rounded upper-body workout.

Like the 'look mum no hands' approach? Then take it to the stepper in IDEA 13, *Stairway to heaven*, and see how your balance holds out there.

Try another idea...

GONNA GET ELLIPTICAL ON YO' ASS

Of course the whole point of the elliptical trainer is that it's not just upper; your lower body muscles are working merrily away as well. Here too you can mix and match by backing up – because sometimes the way forwards is to go backwards. The smooth elliptical action makes it easy to go into reverse and walk backwards, which then reverses the action on your muscles and works your buttocks more than your thighs. Again try five minutes of each, switching between the two for a more complete body workout.

'Physical fitness is not only one of the most important keys to a healthy body, it is the basis of a dynamic and creative intellectual activity.'
JOHN F. KENNEDY

Defining idea...

How did
it go?

Q   I tried it but I get very tired very fast.

A   *First check that you've got the machine on a low resistance setting, then focus on your rhythm – this should be more like skiing than running, with a smooth swooping movement of arms and legs. Go with the machine rather than fighting it.*

Q   The guy next to me seems happy working out on maximum resistance, but if I have it only halfway up the scale it becomes so hard I can barely keep it moving.

A   *First off, don't worry about others – you do your workout and let them do theirs, but do bear in mind that with a weight-bearing exercise (like this one) a larger person's weight, if they know how to use the rhythm and momentum, will help them overcome the resistance.*

Q   I like it but what's the best setting for fat burning?

A   *Relatively slow and steady is the answer – from 65 to 75 per cent of your maximum heart rate. If your gym has one of the elliptical trainers that incorporates a stride counter, then try keeping it at around 120–130 strides per minute with bursts of 140–160.*

19

Roman revenge

You want a Britney Belly or a Stallone Six-Pack but you're already crunching till you puke and that rock-hard belly is stubbornly refusing to show. How do you make that difference?

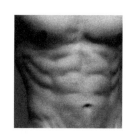

Abs, as they say, are made in the kitchen, not in the gym. Which is largely true — for most of us the problem with getting a muscular midriff is not the muscles, it's the layer of fat sitting on top of them and spoiling the view.

That said, what if you succeed in burning away that fat only to find that the muscles underneath are more washout than washboard? Most gym goers who've been watching their navels are already familiar with, and heartily sick of, the crunch, so what else is there to work the abs? Time for the torture apparatus.

ROMAN WHAT?

Roman chairs come in a variety of shapes but they all look distinctly uncomfortable and have two basic features in common. The first is a padded bar to tuck your lower legs under, and the second is a larger pad to take the weight of your lower body

Here's an idea for you... **Roman chair not tough enough for you? Do you find yourself swaggering up to it with a sneer on your face? OK, you're ready to go up a gear. Next time, instead of having your hands on your ears as you crunch/hyperextend, try having them folded across your chest – holding a weight. Remember to take it steady at first – no grunting away with a 50 kg plate on your chest – but as you build up the load so you will build up the muscle.**

(bum or groin, depending which way up you're facing). There may be other bits and bobs to the chair in your gym – it may be at a 45 degree angle, or have handles, or a flat foot-plate, but these are mere frills and frippery.

NOW WHAT DO I DO?

There are two basic ways of using the chair: face down, which gives you a great back hyperextension (and an unrivalled view of the floor), and face up, which also gives you a great back hyperextension (and an unrivalled view of the ceiling).

Notice that word 'hyperextension'. The point of the Roman chair is that it makes your muscles work through a wider range of movement than usual, and if you have a weak back this could be dangerous. *If in doubt, take professional advice.*

Make sure you're nicely warmed up and then assume the position. Lie face down, with the backs of your calves tucked under the padded bar, your elbows bent and your hands on your ears. Now smoothly bend your body forwards and extend your shoulders down towards the floor. Equally smoothly bring your body back to horizontal, and then arch upwards so you are lifting your shoulders and chest high off the horizontal. This will work your back muscles but you will also quickly realise that you have to tense your stomach muscles (and your buttocks) to maintain the position. That's a rep. Try ten to twelve more.

Crunch fanatics looking to add a little more zest to their routine can also flip the other way up, and lock their feet under the bar with their bum on the pad. Now crunch as normal. The difference is that because there's no floor under your back you have to keep tense all the time with no respite.

Like the idea of varying your abs routine but uncomfortable with the chair (or unsure your back is up to this?) Try the hanging leg lifts described in IDEA 20, *Hanging around.*

Try another idea...

For killer obliques turn sideways on the chair and extend down and up. Don't attempt the same range of movement as you would face down as you won't make it and it will be very intense.

'What did the Romans ever do for us?'
From Monty Python's *Life of Brian.*

Defining idea...

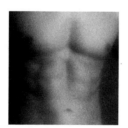

Q **I asked if there was a Roman chair and they pointed to an upright frame with elbow pads. Has one of us lost the plot?**

A *Strictly speaking the Roman chair is the stripped-down bench described here. Because it uses the same muscles some gyms refer to the apparatus for hanging leg raises as the Roman chair. To learn how to hang a leg raise, have a look at IDEA 20, Hanging around.*

Q **I'm finding it hard to even do ten reps. Can I make it easier?**

A *Try changing your arm position. If having your hands on your ears is too hard, then fold your arms across your chest or even hold your arms straight down your sides as you do the move.*

Q **I'm fine on doing those ten reps now – do I have to start clutching weight plates if I want to make it any harder?**

A *No, you can make life just a smidgen more sweaty simply by extending your arms out straight above your head.*

Q **I see other people doing sit ups on the Roman chair sitting on the pad, with their toes hooked under the foot bar. Should I give this a go?**

A *In a word, no. If you're looking to work your abs, then sit-ups of any kind are less efficient because your abs only take care of the first part of the lifting movement. After that they're aided by the psoas muscle which helps haul you up to the sitting position. Of course this means that you're developing a great psoas muscle, but since the psoas runs from the top of your thigh bones through the pelvic girdle to your spine, only a surgeon is ever going to admire it.*

20

Hanging around
– hanging abs workout

Summer's coming, and the siren call of the swimsuit means you're stealing nervous peeks at your belly. You've done everything you can to strip the fat off, but what's left underneath isn't quite the toned midsection you see on MTV. What to do?

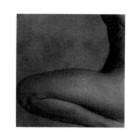

There comes a point when the revelation dawns that crunches, splendid as they are, may not be the whole answer.

That point usually comes when you realise that you can do forty or more of the things, and with any other weight-bearing exercise you'd have upped the weight by now to make it more difficult. Well here's how to up the weight, and vary your routine in the process – all by hanging around in the gym.

WHAT DO I NEED?

Hanging leg raises can be performed from a chinning bar (the horizontal metal bar set above head height) but unless you have a grip like a second-hand car salesman you'll find it very tiring on the hands. Much better is to look around for a leg-raise 'chair' – sometimes called a Roman chair, but not to be confused with the mutant

Here's an idea for you...

Standard leg raises (bent or straight leg) primarily work the abs (rectus abdominus) but with a twist they can also work the obliques that run down the side of your stomach. Try the bent knees lift as normal but as you raise your leg twist your body to the side so that at the end of the movement your feet are sideways on and perpendicular to the floor. Lower gently back to resting position and do the same movement but for the other side. Resist the temptation to swing your legs up.

bench of the same name (see IDEA 19, *Roman revenge*). The leg-raise chair is a vertical metal frame with a cushioned backrest and support pads to rest your forearms on as they take the weight of your body (your legs hanging freely below). There are usually handles at the end of the forearm pads which both help you get a grip and push slightly against so that your back is set snugly into the cushioned backrest.

WHAT DO I DO?

Having warmed up on something that works upper and lower body (such as an elliptical trainer or a rowing machine), jump up into the chair with your back pressed against the back rest and your weight on your forearms. Step off the foot rests so that your legs are hanging unsupported, then smoothly bend and lift your legs up towards your chest. At the end of the move you should also be tilting your pelvis upwards to get the last part of the lift nice and high. Keeping the whole movement slow and controlled, lower the legs back down to the starting position. That's a rep, try eight to ten more, and see if you can build up from one set of ten to three or four.

To make it harder you can try the exercise with 'straight' legs but don't lock the knees and try to keep them slightly bent. If you're swinging your legs up from the hip to raise them, then you're probably doing wonders for your hip flexors but you won't be working your abs properly. Keep it smooth and controlled at all times, and don't ignore any tightness or strain in your back.

Try another idea...

If you're looking for new ways to mould your midsection, then you might want to take a look at IDEAS 11 and 12, *Balls I* and *Balls II*. If you're looking for tougher ways to tone, then try IDEA 19, *Roman revenge*.

Defining idea...

'I have flabby thighs, but fortunately my stomach covers them.'
JOAN RIVERS

How did it go?

Q **Even with legs bent I can only manage a couple of these. Should I give up and go back to normal crunches?**

A *As long as the problem is lack of strength and not pain from your back then persevere, but try this version. Start with your knees completely bent and pulled up so that your thighs are horizontal with the ground. Now just use your pelvis to tilt upwards towards your chest for a moment. Lower, and repeat.*

Q **It went well but I can already do the straight leg raise and I'm looking for a variation to make it tougher. What's next?**

A *Try the leg-lift. With one leg straight, bend the other so the ankle crosses the first leg just above the knee. Slightly bend the supporting leg to take the pressure off your back and now raise that leg up as if you were doing a straight leg lift – only this time the working leg is also lifting the crossed leg. That should make things interesting for you.*

Q **And if I want to work my obliques harder?**

A *Try oblique scissors. Starting off with your body twisted sideways, slightly bend both your legs. Now lift the outside leg (that's the right if you're twisted with your right shoulder outwards) up to as close to horizontal with the ground as you can, leaving the other leg in the down position. Next lift the second leg to join the first. Smoothly lower the second leg, then the first to join it. That's a rep.*

21

At a stretch

Stretching seems like a pain, so when time is tight it's probably the first thing to drop off your workout to-do list. Skip the stretching, however, and you increase the injury risk and miss out on sports performance.

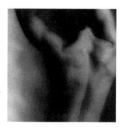

Skipping the stretching is one of those naughty little sins we've all been guilty of from time to time.

Stretching takes time, it's uncomfortable and it's hard to see the point. Until something goes wrong of course, at which point you can't decide which is harder to put up with – your pulled/torn/slipped thingumajig, or all that told-you-so stuff about stretching from your trainer/chiropractor/doctor. Bizarre though it sounds, it's possible that the time you're spending in the gym may be just setting you up for an injury. Strength training creates stronger muscles but may reduce the flexibility of the connective tissue surrounding the muscle groups. Which means that the fitter you are, the more you need to stretch.

There's more to stretching than just avoiding injury, however. By gently extending the range of movement in joints and muscles you open up new performance possibilities. Longer strides when running, or strokes when swimming, and better skiing technique are among the potential benefits of extended flexibility.

Here's an idea for you...

The three-way stretch is so called because it stretches your back, arms and hamstring all in one. Sit on the floor with one leg straight out in front of you. Bend the other leg, pulling your ankle as far up into your groin as you can with the sole of your foot resting on upper thigh of the other leg. Now with both hands reach down the straight leg as far as you can. If you can reach your toes then hold them, if not don't strain yourself. Try not to tense the straight leg. You should feel the stretch right across your back and down the back of your leg (hamstring). Hold for thirty seconds, gently release and switch legs.

Before you start stretching there are a couple of old ideas you need to bury once and for all. Back at school all we were likely to be taught about stretching was some nonsense about touching your toes and 'bouncing' the stretch to reach further. This approach belongs back in the days when people doing exercise wore full-length stripy swimming costumes and sported handlebar moustaches. Bouncing a stretch is likely to tear or strain something – precisely the opposite of the purpose here. Forget all that Jane Fonda era 'no pain, no gain' nonsense as well – *if it hurts, stop it at once.*

Stretch steadily, and stretch often, easing into a stretch only to that delicate point where it's edging on discomfort and absolutely not to the point where it hurts to hold the stretch. You may have heard of ballistic stretching which is highly athletic and active. You may also have heard of BASE jumping, crocodile wrestling and skeleton luge but it doesn't mean you have to do them. Leave ballistic stretches to others, just focus on nice static work for the moment.

Your muscles should be warm when you stretch (don't confuse stretching and warming up) and you should hold the stretch for thirty seconds with up to a minute tops if you're very comfortable. Although the temptation is to head for the shower as soon as you get off the treadmill/stepper/bike it is precisely at that moment, when you're still hot and bothered, that stretching can do the most good.

The most common stretches are…

You like the idea of a longer, leaner, less injury-prone you? Then take a look at IDEA 36, *Piling on the Pilates.*

Try another idea…

Quadriceps – Standing upright, balance on one leg and bend the other so you can catch the foot in your hand. Flex it gently back up to your buttocks. Very slightly bend the knee of the leg you're balancing on and tip the hips forward to feel the stretch down the front of your thigh. Hold for thirty seconds, gently go back to standing and switch legs.

Calves – Stand four or five steps away from and facing a wall. Now keeping your left foot in the original position place your right foot halfway between you and the wall and reach forward with your outstretched arms so you're leaning against the wall with your hands. Your right leg should now be bent and your left leg straight out behind you with the sole of the foot flat on the floor. Feel the stretch up the back of the calf for thirty seconds, gently go back to standing and switch legs.

Triceps – Reach one arm straight up above your head then bend it at the elbow so your hand is now behind your neck. Reach up with the other hand, take the first elbow, and gently pull it down and across in the direction of the pulling arm's shoulder. Hold, release, switch.

'*I must be right. Never an aspirin. Never injured a day in my life. The whole country, the whole world, should be doing my exercises. They'd be happier.*'
JOSEPH H. PILATES

Defining idea…

Shoulder – Hold your arm out straight in front of you, then move it across your body, placing the other hand on the upper arm between elbow and shoulder. Use that hand to push the arm in towards the chest. Hold, release, switch.

There's a stretch for every part of your body – including a few you're probably not familiar with yet. Take the time to find out about the stretches specific to your sport, and then take the time to do them.

How did it go?

Q   I feel too stiff to get into the positions you mention. Is it possible that I'm just not flexible enough to do them?

A   *It's possible that you're a little too inflexible now, but stretching is the answer not the problem. Don't worry if your stretch isn't as spectacular as others – just push it to the point where you can feel it, without it being painful.*

Q   There's a stretching class at my gym. Should I go?

A   *Absolutely. Properly done, a stretching class is an excellent way to learn new techniques and can be very relaxing. Men tend to shy away from them, but then men are also far more likely to end up injured. One word of advice though – timetable pressures mean that few classes have enough time to warm up thoroughly, so spend twenty minutes on an exercise machine warming up on your own prior to the class.*

Q   You warn about the danger of confusing stretching and warming up. Does that mean I should never stretch before exercise?

A   *No, just that you should never stretch when your muscle is cold. Stretching before working muscles for your principal exercise is a good idea, as long as you have done enough activity to warm them up. Remember we're talking about warming up that specific muscle here, not just about getting generally warmed up.*

22

Explode into action – the power of plyometrics

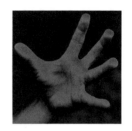

Sudden explosive bursts of power are what make the memorable moments in so many sports. Plyometrics can give you the edge for those sporting moments – the jump, the kick or the serve – that can make all the difference on the day.

Plyometrics aren't for everyone — not least because their explosive nature means they entail a higher risk of injury than most other exercises.

What they can do, however, is prepare you for those fleeting seconds of all-or-nothing effort. Whether your goal is that winning judo throw, an awesome kick or the speed spurt that leaves tacklers and rivals clutching at empty air, you'll need to train for bursts of power. Enter plyometrics.

The idea behind plyometrics is much like that of a spring. The more you 'load' a spring by pushing down on it, the higher it bounces back when you let go. Similarly you can 'load' a muscle by contracting it 'eccentrically', by lengthening it, then immediately contracting it 'concentrically' (by shortening it). The idea is that you

If standing jumps are too simple for your taste, try step jumps. Set up a step (borrow one from the step class) so that it's about a foot high. Step backwards off the top of it so you drop to the ground, then immediately bounce back up to land on the step. If you step backwards, then the jump will be forwards. If the step is stable enough you can step off forwards and jump back backwards. If you want to vary that a little more, set up two steps a couple of feet apart and step forwards off one to bounce up onto the other before reversing the motion to end up where you started.

get a boost in the force of the second contraction. If it sounds like hard work, that's because it is, and because it involves a double contraction in such a short period of time it is very demanding and only to be considered by those already in very good shape. There are a few other sensible precautions to take with plyometrics:

Always warm up thoroughly. Cold muscles are the most likely to tear at any time. Start shocking them with load and explosive release and you increase that risk.

Don't do plyometrics after a strength workout when the muscles are already tired. Remember that sprinting is already a plyometric workout, so attempting lower-body plyometrics (like jumping) after a sprint or interval session is courting fatigue or worse.

Keep the volume low. OK, so you can do forty press-ups on one arm, but that doesn't mean you can do ten with a clap thrown in. Plyometric sets mean six to ten reps. If you're doing jumps, then start at around fifty jumps per session as a maximum (count landings – that's what your spine is doing) and work up to a hundred – gently.

Give yourself plenty of rest between sessions. These exercises are very intensive so two sessions a week should be your maximum.

Cushion the fall. Wear proper sports shoes, avoid concrete floors and don't do plyometric press-ups without a mat to land on.

Starting to feel the burn of sudden jumps? Why not try a step class (IDEA 15, *Stepping up a gear*).

Try another idea...

LOWER BODY

Standing jump – Stand with your feet shoulder-width apart. Squat down slightly and immediately explode upwards, reaching both arms up for the ceiling (brownie points if you touch it). Take care to land with knees slightly bent to cushion the shock.

Side jump – Start as for the standing jump but this time jump sideways about a foot, landing both feet together. Immediately bounce back again.

'There's only one way to think about this game and one way to play it. That's all out, foot to the floor, pushing myself as hard as I can for as long as I can.'
'MAGIC' JOHNSON

Defining idea...

UPPER BODY

Clap press-up – The first time you try this you'll think the above is a spelling mistake. Take up the normal press-up position, drop down fast, then push up so hard you lift up off the ground, clap your hands together in the air, then get them back into the original position fast enough to catch yourself on the ground. Repeat.

Sideways throw – Take a heavy but bouncy ball (football or basketball – a rugby ball would be showing off) and stand few feet away from a solid wall with your side towards the wall and your feet shoulder-width apart. Hold the ball in front of you in both hands and twist first away from the wall then swing back the other way releasing the ball at the wall with enough force that it bounces back into your hands. As soon as you've caught it you should be swinging back the other way. This is good for co-ordination, as well as working those obliques and abs.

Q I'm practising side jumps but finding it hard to know if I'm jumping far or high enough to make any real difference. Any ideas?

A If you want to make this more challenging, try to position an obstacle to jump back and forth over. Something about mid-calf height should do it. Preferably something less solid than you are should you fail to clear it.

Q How can I be sure I'm giving it my all in vertical jumps?

A If you're tall you could always try doing them under a basketball hoop and touch the net (or rim if you're that tall) each time. Otherwise find or visualise a mark on a wall that you can jump up to the first time you do the exercise and try not to fall short of it on each consecutive jump.

Q I've tried the clap press-up and it lives up to its (near) name. I can barely do one or two – how can I get better without flattening my nose on the floor in the process?

A Simple. Try doing the same thing but without the clap – just focus on bouncing yourself up in the air at the top of each press up and then drop back down into the next one.

23

Getting groovy with the Gravitron

It sounds like something Luke Skywalker would drive to work in, but get to know it and you'll find that the Gravitron is as clever as it is big when it comes to upper-body workouts.

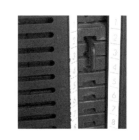

I once asked a personal trainer what his favourite piece of gym equipment was and he pointed to something that looked like an accident in a girder factory and sighed like someone remembering their first love. At the time I think I edged away quietly and avoided him for quite some while.

But I was wrong, and he was right. The heap of scaffolding that had won his heart was the Gravitron machine and if you're interested in upper-body strength and toning, then to know the Gravitron is to love it.

Here's an idea for you...

If you really want to make life tough for yourself, try pull-ups with a towel grip. You may want to counterbalance yourself with more weight than usual as this is much tougher. You'll need two small sweat towels. Drape a towel over each upper hand rest and take firm hold of the ends so you're gripping the hanging towel ends not the bar. Now try to pull up. As you may have noticed this also uses the gripping muscles of the hand and wrist. And how.

The idea is simple. Working with your own bodyweight is a great way of building strength and hauling yourself up and down is a natural movement that combines many muscles at once. There's just one catch. It's all very well singing the praises of pull-ups (or chin-ups – call them what you will) and dips, but we're not all built like marines, and some of us struggle to complete a single rep. On any other weight-lifting exercise the answer would be to lower the weight and work at an easier level until we got stronger. Working with your own bodyweight, however, makes this a tad tricky since shedding our own pounds means more than just slotting a pin into a different figure. Which is where the Gravitron comes in.

The Gravitron works by the same sort of weights and pulleys as all the other weights machines, except that here they are set up as counterbalances acting against your bodyweight. Which means that the more weight you select on the Gravitron, the less weight you actually have lift to get your body to perform dips and pull-ups. You get the same range of movement as the real thing, but you get to choose just how hard it is to do. Perfect.

There are two basic exercises:

Dips – The triceps and shoulder exercise *par excellence*, dips tone those upper arms a treat. Although people tend to fuss over their biceps, it's the triceps that make up two-thirds of your upper arm muscle.

If you like the idea of using weights but don't want to stray into the weights room, then read a little more about pump classes in IDEA 33, *Pump that body.*

Try another idea...

First, set a weight on the Gravitron. Remember that however many kilos it says on the metal plate you select, the figure you will lift is your weight minus that figure. The more weight you select, the easier it is for you to complete the exercise.

Now kneel on the knee pads facing the machine and hold the lower set of hand grips which should be at about waist level. Smoothly lower your body by bending your elbows until your upper arms are parallel with the floor. Straighten your arms to return to your original position. That's a rep.

Pull-ups – The pull-up has a bit of an image as a hard man's exercise which makes it all the better watching grannies doing it on the

'*Don't get sand kicked in your face.*'
CHARLES ATLAS

Defining idea...

Gravitron. The principal muscles worked are the lats of your back, and the biceps as you bend your arms in the last part of the pull. You start exactly as for the dips, but this time reach up for the bars above your head. Pull up until your head reaches at least hand level and let yourself slowly back down. That's a rep.

How did
it go?

**Q   There's a choice of grips on the pull-up bars of the Gravitron.
Should I go for the wider or the narrower grip?**

A   *The idea behind the different grips is that the wider you have your grip, the
more you are using the 'lats' of your back to complete the action, and the
narrower your grip, the more you help them out with the biceps. Since half
the point of a combination workout like this is to work out lots of muscles I
suggest you mix and match so as to keep your muscles on their toes.*

**Q   I can't help but notice that on the fixed pull-up bar in the free
weights room there are large men hauling their whole bodies very
fast up and down. With the Gravitron it's hard to do it so fast – is
this a good thing?**

A   *Yes. Macho pressure means that the temptation in public is to do as many
lifts as possible, regardless of form. High speed often means that people
are using momentum and probably swinging their hips and legs to achieve
the lift. Your steady progress on the Gravitron will give you a more thorough
upper-body workout.*

**Q   If I get to the point where I have no weight selected on the
Gravitron is that the same as an unassisted dip/pull-up on the old-
fashioned bars?**

A   *Nearly. To nit-pick there is still some resistance from the pulleys and the
mechanism itself which in the case of the Gravitron are working for your.
Still, if you're confident that you don't need any counterbalance, then
maybe it's time to try on the normal bars. Just don't lose that good form
that the Gravitron imposes on you.*

24
Meeting Mr Smith

The Smith machine is an intimidating lump of metal, but get to grips with it and you'll find it offers a far more forgiving path into working with weights than the conventional approach of barbells and bruises.

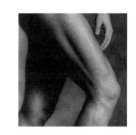

If the Smith machine could get up and slope off down the pub it would probably sit at the bar and whine to the barmaid about how misunderstood it is.

Neither fish nor fowl, it larks somewhere between weight machines and full-on free weights. Newcomers to weights tend to be put off both by its bulk, and by those intimidating weight plates that have to be loaded onto it. Body builders positively queue up to pour scorn on it for not involving the full range of motion of a barbell. There again, it's in the nature of newcomers to be nervous of anything new, and as for body builders…let's not forget that there are body builders out there who wouldn't flinch at the thought of pumping themselves full of elephant laxative if they thought it would make part of them swell up more.

Meanwhile for those of us who at least inhabit the same galaxy as Planet Normal the Smith machine may look like full on 'iron' but feels much more like the kind of machines we're already used to.

All the above presume you don't have time for benchwork, but if you do, then the Smith comes into its own. Either set up a flat bench and try bench pressing without the need for a spotter's help, or set it up as an incline seat (so the 'back' of the chair slopes backwards) and do incline chest presses. By working at an incline you shift the load onto the shoulders and upper chest.

The Smith machine (invented by a Mr Smith, surprise surprise) is basically a barbell trapped in a metal frame so that it can only move straight up and down in a smooth sliding motion. It has hooks on the bar so it can be locked into different resting positions at different heights. To load it you slide weight plates onto the ends. To work with it you can set it on a high starting position and stand underneath it for squats or lunges where your legs are doing the work of raising the weight. Alternatively you can position a bench under it and work sitting down, for example doing military presses where you push a weight up from your shoulders to the point where your arms are straight. Another position is to use the bench lying down and bench press your little heart out.

Its critics are right – because the bar only moves in one direction and one plane you won't develop all the stabilising muscles used for free weights. So serious body builders should stick to barbells. But the Smith machine allows us normal mortals to feel much safer using weights because we don't have to worry about becoming unbalanced. Or squashed like a pancake – those hooks on the bar mean that you don't need a 'spotter' to grab the weight and stop you getting flattened if you get overambitious. Simply turning your wrists engages the hook on the next rest point down the rack. If the weight suddenly feels like too much, then a quick twist of the wrist hands it back to the care of Mr Smith.

The Smith machine is not a place to start learning about weights from scratch. If terms like 'bench press', 'squats' or 'lunges' have you furrowing your brow in confusion, then ask an instructor for help or better yet try a pump class.

If you're already comfortable with the basic lifts, however, try the following with the helping hand of Mr Smith to steady you.

In a hurry? No bench? No problem.

Squat – Start with feet shoulder-width apart, bar resting on shoulders, knees very slightly bent (never locked). Gently lower down as if trying to sit (never drop as low as full sitting position) and then back up again – great for thighs. Then...

Bend over row – With the bar starting at between knee and hip height, feet shoulder-width apart, bend over the bar and lift it by pulling your elbows up to shoulder level. Works the lats (back), shoulders and arms. Then...

Lunges – Split stance (one leg forward, one back) with bar on shoulders. Lower (rear leg bends) and raise by pushing up with the forward leg. Another killer for leg muscles and a good one on the Smith because it forces you to move the weight straight up and down. Then...

Incline push-ups – Lock the bar on the lowest setting and assume the press up position but with your hands on the bar, not the floor. Press-ups should be easier than they are on the horizontal so go for more than you would normally. Good for triceps and chest.

If you're new to weights but want strength and toning, then try a pump class (see IDEA 33, *Pump that body*). which will teach you all the favourite moves and give you an all-round workout with light weights.

Try another idea...

'Start wide, expand further, and never look back.'
ARNOLD SCHWARZENEGGER

Defining idea...

How did it go?

Q **When I lunge it's the leg behind me that feels it the most with an almost unbearable tenseness. What am I doing wrong?**

A   *Check your body position. In a lunge the weight should be lifted by the bent (forward) leg and your quads should do the work. Check that you are starting squarely under the bar, not with it slightly behind your shoulders.*

Q **I've heard that squats damage your knees – is this true?**

A   *There are cases of knee damage due to overenthusiastic or misguided squatting, but the Smith machine reduces the chance of damage due to unbalance. If you are in any doubt, then you're probably using too much weight.*

Q **I like the idea but the weights for the machine are too big for me to lift comfortably. Any suggestions?**

A   *Try it without weights at all – the machine resistance and the weight of the bar itself are calculated to weigh around 7–10 kg (depending on the model) so even with no plates on you're still lifting weight.*

25
Take it slow

In a hurry to get stronger? *Slow down*. That's the promise of super slow lifting, a technique that promises better results from fewer repetitions and only one or two sessions a week.

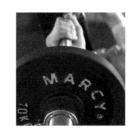

Some people just love hanging around in weight rooms but most of us just want to do our stuff and get out of there. Besides, we have lives and stuff.

Or so we like to think. So how about a strength routine that demands just one set of just six or eight repetitions, and only needs one or two sessions a week? Advocates of this approach also promise greater strength gains than traditional weight training. So what's the trick? Simple, while all the other boys and girls are haring through their strength sessions, you save real time with fewer lifts at a truly tortoise-like tempo.

Taking it slowly is not to be confused with taking it easy. The approach requires only a few lifts, but each one takes 15–20 seconds consisting of a slow lift, hold and slow descent. Try it and you'll find that seconds have never crawled past so slowly. You'll certainly feel your muscles though. Super slow lifting has attracted a sect-like following of true believers who swear that slowing it down is vastly superior to

Here's an idea for you...

If you've tried slow lifting and found you like it, the normal route onwards and upwards would be to increase the weight you use and perform the same number of reps. Try working to muscle failure instead. Keep going on a weight, just as slowly, until you realise you simply aren't going to manage to lift it all the way for ten seconds. In keeping with the technique, however, remember not to just drop it – even if you can't make the full lift, you should try to slow down the descent just as much as usual.

speeding it up. Fitness fanatics being what they are, however, there is an equal and opposite movement that claims that the benefits are only in the early stages of strength training and don't help the hardcore. So if you've got arms like legs and muscles on your muscles, don't bother to read on. But if you're fairly new to strength training, short of time or looking for something different, then note that whatever the argument about gains for the long-term trainer, the short-term benefits are:

- Yes, slow lifting does give a more intensive session within a shorter time.

- Even the purists admit that it does teach good form as you have to focus on each part of the lift.

- It takes momentum out of the equation so you can't 'cheat' by swinging your way through a set.

- It's less likely to cause injuries through jerky technique.

Which makes slow lifting worth a try, especially if you only get to the weights room once a week.

TRY THIS WORKOUT

Squats – Using a barbell, squat machine or Smith machine (see IDEA 24, *Meeting Mr Smith*) try a weight you can normally lift comfortably 12–20 times and try for six to eight lifts counting ten seconds up, ten seconds down. That's a rep. Six or seven more of those and that's a wrap.

Bench press – As above, preferably using a Smith machine unless you are confident you can stabilise a barbell for such a long lift (and you have a spotter to watch over you).

Having tried the technique on larger muscles, try it with smaller muscle groups or even individual muscles such as:

■ Shoulder press
■ Preacher curl (biceps)
■ Triceps press.

For the exact opposite of super slow, take a look at the pump class in IDEA 33, *Pump that body*.

Try another idea...

'*In a nutshell, SuperSlow® is raising the weight in ten seconds and lowering the weight in ten seconds. There are minor exceptions to this, but this is the basic plan. If you perform and arm bending movement and time yourself you will see that it is creepy slow.*'
KEN HUTCHINS, high priest of 'creepy slow', and the developer (and patent holder) of the SuperSlow® protocol.

Defining idea...

How did
it go?

Q **I try to count the full ten seconds on the lift and the lower but find I just have to rush through it a little faster, especially on the lower. What am I doing wrong?**

A *It may seem odd, because you're probably using a lighter weight than you're used to, but you've probably overloaded yourself. Decrease the amount of weight until you can perform the full ten second lift and ten second lower – correct form is everything in this exercise.*

Q **I've read that the super slow technique has fat-burning benefits and can even replace aerobic activity. Is this true?**

A *Ken Hutchins, who founded SuperSlow®, made a name for himself by attacking aerobics, and if you've ever seen an 80s exercise video (all big hair and leg-warmers) you may understand. Slow lifting does burn calories, but it is no substitute for cardiovascular exercise. Your heart is still the most important muscle you can 'pump'.*

Q **I just tried the workout and it was hard but I don't feel tired afterwards. Should I try it again with heavier weights?**

A *Steady on there. One of the reasons why you only do one or two sessions a week with super slow is that there is a phenomena by which muscle soreness may not set in for two or even three days. With this technique patience is the key both when working and resting.*

26

Pyramid power

Lifting weights and pushing iron around quickly gets boring – both for you and for your muscles. To keep both you and your body on its toes, try varying the routine a little.

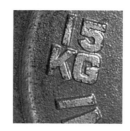

When you were first shown strength training you were probably taught to perform a set of repetitions three or four times at the same weight.

When you could do all that comfortably, you upped the weight a notch. That's been the theory of strength building since the days when Samson used to practice horizontal shoulder presses on pillars. It's a system that works, but that doesn't mean it's the only one, and whether you're trying to tone up or bulk up it pays to vary the routine.

PYRAMID POWER

There's nothing that complicated about pyramid sets. You start with lighter weights and more repetitions, then increase the weights and decrease the repetitions with each set. Starting with 'light and lots' helps stretch and warm the muscles before you hit them with the heavy stuff and so helps prevent injury. Psychologically it also

Here's an idea for you...

The pyramid set described here is really a modification of the true pyramid set beloved by serious weightlifters. For the full pyramid you don't stop with the third set of heavier weights but instead continue back down the pyramid by doing further sets with lighter weights and higher repetitions. Rather than ending up doing five or more sets, try doing the normal pyramid set, ending on your heaviest weights and lifting those to failure (i.e. you can't complete that last lift). Then drop the weight down by a couple of notches and lift ten more of the lighter weight. There you go, that should leave you pretty much good for nothing but the shower.

becomes easier to move up to heavier weights; although each set gets heavier it also involves fewer reps. Us men in particular tend to enjoy pyramid sets because we're forever trying to play with heavier dumbbells or notch the machine up one more number than before. The pyramid system means that the final set is probably using a heavier weight than we could manage in the classic approach (albeit for fewer repetitions), so we get to walk away from the machine feeling well chuffed.

Try this pyramid set with dumbbells – please note that these weights are just for guidance, if you happen to be built like a carthorse then clearly you would need to up the weight.

Try doing curls, standing in front of the mirror, and using a 'hammer' grip so that when your arm is at the top of the lift the weight is vertical in your hand, as if you were holding a hammer. Don't move your upper body or shoulder to help with the exercise.

- Set 1 – 1 kg dumbbell, 12 reps
- Set 2 – 1.5 kg dumbbell, 10 reps
- Set 3 – 2 kg dumbbell, 8 reps

You get the idea. The same principle can be applied to any of the weight machines, the Smith machine or the free weights.

Try another idea...

If you're looking for variety in weight training, or you just don't seem to be getting results from your current workout, try super slow lifting – see IDEA 25, *Take it slow.*

Defining idea...

'For years coaches would not allow athletes to lift weights because it made them look muscle-bound. Now weight training is a main part of almost any team's training programme.'
LOU FERRIGNO, bodybuilder and American football player. (You have to say he also proves the coaches' point though – let's not forget he played 'The Hulk' on TV. Moderation in everything.)

How did it go?

Q **I've been trying the pyramid set for a month or two now. Can I tweak it more for my goal which is pure strength rather than toning?**

A   *Sure. Instead of doing a pyramid of 12–10–8 reps, try a more concentrated pyramid of 10–8–6 reps. Make sure you warm up before this because you are moving into the area of very low rep, high weight work. Dropping the reps below six isn't recommended unless you are very serious about strength work and have taken professional advice.*

Q **I've been using the pyramid set for a while and have moved up my weight on my favourite exercise. The only problem is that while I can complete the twelve and the ten rep sets without trouble, I'm struggling with the eight rep. I'm loathe to drop back down a weight as that seems like admitting defeat.**

A   *Then don't. Cheat a little on the harder weight by doing as many as you can, then resting a moment, then squeezing out another rep, resting a moment, and so on until you complete the eight rep set. Now work on cutting the rest moments down each time until the set is as smooth as the lighter lift sets.*

Q **I like the idea of pyramid sets, but the bulk of my work is done using my own bodyweight – press-ups, dips, pull-ups, etc. Is there any way of applying the pyramid approach to this?**

A   *That depends on your strength at the moment. If you have difficulty completing a set of twelve dips/pull-ups, then try using a Gravitron machine (see IDEA 23, Getting groovy with the Gravitron) which enables you to vary the effort of each rep. If you're already doing full sets of dips/pull-ups, then the only option is to make them harder for the smaller rep 'peak' of the pyramid. Try a small (but sturdy) rucksack with a weight in it.*

27

The muscles that time forgot

We all know what biceps are, and most of us are so convinced of the existence of abs that we spend weeks digging for them. But what about the rhomboids and obliques? Here are a few moves especially for the sinews that slipped your mind.

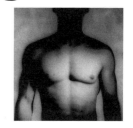

For as long as man (and here, we're talking about man, rather than woman) has built muscle he has obsessed about whatever 'show muscles' are in fashion.

Up until about twenty years ago that mainly meant the almighty biceps, as can be gauged from the fact that otherwise normal males, invited to assume a 'strong' pose will immediately bend their arms and study them intently for some hoped-for swelling. *Baywatch* and a rash of men's physique magazines have seen the biceps tipped off the top spot by the rectus abdominis, *abs* to its friends. The era of the abs has also ushered in sexual equality when it comes to standing nervously in front of the mirror trying to get the jiggly bits to stay still.

For every show horse, however, there is a work horse, a Cinderella muscle that does the drudge work out of sight while the sinews with the good PR hog the limelight and the workout time. Which wouldn't really bother any but the most soft hearted

Here's an idea for you...

Working on stronger arms often focuses on upper arms at the expense of forearm strength. Try wrapping a sweat towel around the bar or hand grips when lifting to make the grip bigger and work the wrist and forearm muscles more.

of us if it wasn't for the fact that from time to time these work horse muscles decide to go on strike. Since so many muscles work in pairs they may even be finding their work harder due to the overdevelopment of their more glamorous partners. So here's a run down of some of the sinews that may have slipped your mind, and a few ideas for how to make sure these Cinderellas have a ball.

YOU CAN POINT TO YOUR ABS...BUT WHAT ABOUT YOUR OBLIQUES, TRANSVERSUS AND ERECTOR SPINAE?

We all want toned tummies, and we've all crunched away like clockwork toys to get them – but the crunch only really works the rectus abdominis muscle (the one that forms the six-pack). To get a really strong midsection, you've also got to pay attention to the external and internal obliques and the transversus abdominis.

The obliques work together down the sides of our abdomen and take care of turning motions. Crunches with a twist (right arm to left knee for example) will work the obliques, or for a bit of variation try this:

Obliques – Swiss ball Russian twist
Sounds like a cocktail but sadly isn't. Sit on a Swiss ball and walk your legs away forwards so that you are left with your hips and lower torso on the ball. Now lift your shoulders up and forwards and with your arms extended straight out like a sleepwalker twist your upper body sideways to the left, to the centre again, then the right. Repeat.

Transversus – abdominal breathing

The transversus lies beneath the other stomach muscles and can't be seen. The effect of it can though, since a strong and taut transversus not only armour plates your midriff but flattens it.

For a workout that doesn't skimp on the smaller muscles try a pump class (see IDEA 33, *Pump that body*).

Try another idea...

Lie flat on your back and place the flat of your hand on your stomach to feel what's going on. Now breath in deeply for a count of four, breathing from your stomach – imagine drawing that diaphragm deep down towards your pelvis. Expel the air for eight counts by compressing your stomach muscles, then hold that muscle pressed against your spine for a minute and try to breathe normally without letting it relax.

Erector spinae – cable row

These are the muscles that pull your spine straight. Overdoing it on the abs can tighten up your stomach and weaken the pull of the erector spinae, leading to back trouble. Rowing machines will help, but if you're looking for a little extra, try a cable row. A cable row will feature a seat, a foot plate and a low pulley with a cable and handle. Set a light weight, sit on the seat and holding the handle in both hands row it back towards you just as you would on a rowing machine (but without the legs). See IDEA 15, *Good morning Superman*.

'Anyone can go into the gym and lift a weight. The trick is using the proper form to make your muscles give you the results you want.'
SHARON BRUNEAU, bodybuilder

Defining idea...

119

YOU WORK YOUR SHOULDERS AND LATS...BUT WHAT ABOUT YOUR TRAPEZIUS AND RHOMBOIDS?

Lateral pull-downs and dips help build up the lats to get that broad V-shape so sought after by weight-room warriors, but in the process many forget all about the trapezius and the rhomboids. The trapezius goes from half-way up your spine, out to your shoulder and back in to your neck. The rhomboids sit between your shoulder blades and the bottom of your neck and are hidden by the trapezius. These muscles combine to pull your shoulder blades back, but perhaps more importantly they balance out the chest muscles and combine to give pain-free poise. If they are too weak, or unbalanced by an overdeveloped chest, then a shoulder injury could be just waiting to happen.

Trapezius and rhomboids – Smith machine shrug

With feet shoulder-width apart and knees very slightly bent, stand over a lightly weighted bar on the Smith machine (see IDEA 24, *Meeting Mr Smith*) set at about groin height. Keeping your arms at your sides and palms facing backwards, lift the bar by shrugging your shoulders upwards. Repeat. The total movement is only a few centimetres but what matters is that you are not using the lats or shoulders to help.

Q   Is the Smith machine the only way to 'shrug'?

A   Not at all. You can do the same thing by holding a dumbbell in each hand and shrugging upwards.

Q   Try as I might, when I breathe abdominally all I do is suck my stomach in, is this right?

A   Just sucking your stomach in will pull the bottom of your rib cage down towards your pelvis and make it hard to breathe. Try fixing on a point half-way between your navel and your groin and place a finger there so you feel it. Take that as your centre of breathing and try to make the muscles there (rather than higher up) the centre of your contraction.

Q   I can't feel anything in my obliques and I've been doing the Russian twist for ages. How do I spice it up?

A   Try holding a medicine ball in your hands as you do it. To combine it with plyometrics, station a friend on one side and throw the ball to her as you turn, then catch it as she throws it back.

How did it go?

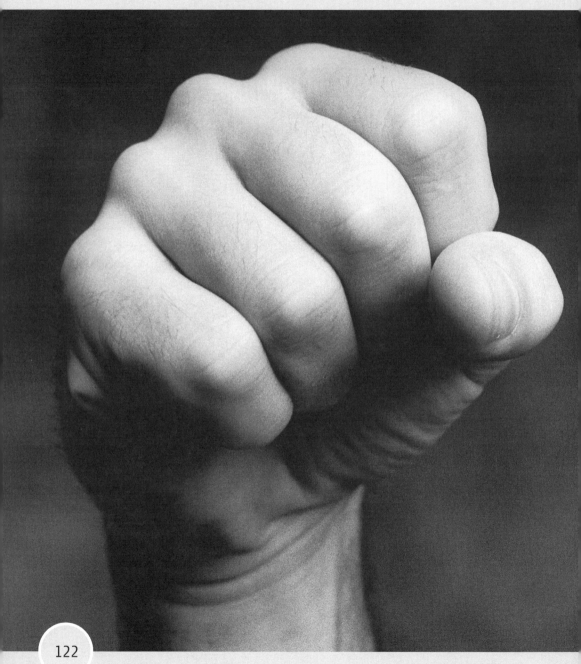

28

Try a tri

Triathlons are deservedly popular as an all-round workout but seem to need a lot of organisation, kit and time. Doing your own in the gym, however, is easy, convenient and doesn't even have to involve getting wet.

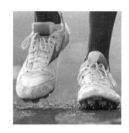

Triathlon is one of the big growth sports of the last ten years, even popping up in the Olympics, and it's not hard to see why.

Unlike traditional long-distance events, triathlon breaks up the race into three disciplines that work different parts of the body in different ways. Triathlons also come in different distances, from the demented (ironman) to the positively bite-sized (super sprint). Even the shortest ones can seem off-putting to newcomers though, since they entail owning/transporting bicycles, and the controlled panic of transitions from one leg to the next. Many triathlons also involve open water swimming – itself enough to make a lot of us nervous. The wonders of the gym, however, mean you can not only try a tri, but compete against your friends, all without buying equipment, or even having to swim.

WHAT DISTANCE?

The full Olympic triathlon distance is a 1.5 km swim, a 40 km cycle and a 10 km run, but most people start with either a 'sprint' distance of 750 m swim, 20 km cycle and

If your gym doesn't have a pool, or you're not comfortable swimming, then simply substitute the rowing machine for the swim. There is even a well-known triathlon that does exactly that. The rower's revenge triathlon starts on a rowing machine before charging outdoors for the ride and run. The rower's revenge distance is 4000 m on a Concept II rowing machine, a 25 km cycle and 7.5 km run.

5 km run, or even a 'super sprint' which is half that distance again. The smart advice says start small and work upwards.

WHAT ORDER?

For safety reasons the swim always comes first (to avoid the risk of tired athletes cramping up in deep water, sometimes known as drowning) but for your indoor triathlon you may want to make the swim last as a way of cooling down. It's still a good idea to do the cycle before the run as it's an efficient and non-impact way of warming up.

WHAT DO I DO?

Having decided your distance, you now have to complete it. First off will be the stationary bike for the distance you have set. Make a note of the time taken but also the resistance level as it will be useful for comparing your performance in the future.

In triathlon the transition times are counted as part of the event, leading to serious scrambles to change clothing and mount/dismount bikes. In the gym that would prove risky so don't include transition times, but do try to go from one activity to the next as fast as you can. The whole point of multisport races is not just how well you do in each individual leg, but how well you perform in the later ones having already put the effort in earlier.

After the bike should come the treadmill. Since you're already nicely warmed up you can get stuck in at your normal running speed for the distance you've set yourself. If you're doing this as a way of working up to the real thing you may want to set the incline to 1 per cent to make up for the lack of wind resistance that you would meet in the open air. Again note your time and the incline you used, then off to the changing rooms and into the pool.

If you fancy a go at triathlon remember that the longest event in it is the bike ride. To get into the swing of competitive cycling without leaving the comfort and warmth of your gym try a spinning class – see IDEA 46, *In a spin*.

Try another idea...

Triathlon swimmers race freestyle (i.e. front crawl) but the rules allow any kind of stroke so don't feel obliged to crawl unless that's what you're comfortable with. This is your triathlon: if you declare that the swimming will be doggy paddle, wearing a life ring and floral bathing cap, then those are the rules.

Once you've completed your first triathlon you might want to think about racing some friends. They don't have to be there with you – as long as you trust each other sufficiently for the honour system to apply. Triathletes often arrange gym triathlons against each other in winter, or when their favourite rivals happen to live in different countries and time zones. Of course the more serious the triathlete, the less reliable the honour system.

'If God invented marathons to keep people from doing anything more stupid, triathlon must have taken Him completely by surprise.'
Triathlete adage, attributed to one P. Z. PEARCE M.D., sports medic

Defining idea...

How did it go?

Q   I realise that for my own tri I can swim any way I like, but I want to work up to the real thing. Do I have to swim front crawl?

A   You can swim any stroke (or mixture of strokes) in triathlon. In any sprint and most Olympic distance races there are usually a few who stick to breast-stroke and they usually beat the odd front-crawler in the process. It's up to you, though do note that backstroke is pretty much unheard of in open water triathlon because of the difficulty of seeing where you're going.

Q   I seem to be getting way faster in my bike leg – suspiciously so. Does the resistance setting on the bike affect the speed?

A   Yes, stationary bikes are unrealistic in the way they clock up speed/distance. Many of them decide you're going much faster if you up the resistance. That's why you'll need to make a note of the level each time and if you race others you may want to agree a resistance level and stick to it.

Q   A friend (in a different gym) and I are getting quite tasty at this triathlon lark but they claim I have the advantage because the pool in my gym is shorter. Any truth in this?

A   'Fraid so. People do record faster times in shorter pools because of the effect of pushing off from the ends.

29

Stepping up a gear

The choreography and clothing of step may look daunting but get over that and give it a try. Step is a full-on cardio workout to music that firms the thighs, shapes the bum and hones the hamstrings.

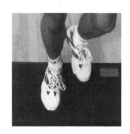

If you've ever peeked in at a step class in action you could well have imagined yourself back in the 80s exercise hell of leotards, leg warmers and shrieking about 'feeling the burn'.

This is a shame since it means that a lot of women, and almost all men, decide on the spot that they are either too uncoordinated, too unfit, too well-dressed or simply too male to take part in the choreographed stampede of a step class.

When step was first introduced it was billed as 'the workout with muscle'. Unlike all that aerobics skipping around that went before it, step introduced high repetition strength moves. This also made it slightly more acceptable to men and it fitted in well with the new man of the 90s who realised that women tended to be more interested in a well-turned buttock than a hairy back and the kind of cleavage shown when builders bend over.

Here's an idea for you...

As you get used to step it gets easier, much easier, which also reduces the benefits of the workout. Most gyms have several levels of step to help keep you on your toes, and you should progress to the next one (intermediate or advanced) as appropriate. In practice, that means as soon as you find that you know what move comes next, you're not as breathless or sweaty as you used to be, or you just fancy something new. Remember, if the new class is too much for you, then simply skip some of the moves to keep up – you'll get it in the end.

Steps of any kind are a surprisingly hard workout – just ask anyone who doesn't live and work in a bungalow. Stepping up and down for an hour is a thorough cardio workout and is only made possible by a careful mix of different moves and motivating music. There's something oddly satisfying in the tap-tap-thud routine akin to, but marginally less embarrassing than, line dancing. Spend a few minutes watching a step class of regulars, everyone beat perfect, stomping their way through their favourite numbers and you'll witness a semi-mystical rite more normally associated with shamans and dervishes.

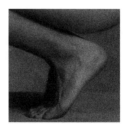

WHAT CAN I EXPECT?

Make sure you start with a beginners' class: step is hard enough work without the stress of playing catch-up. You'll probably warm up with some nice simple side-to-side movements, a bit of stretching as you sway, and some step up/downs. Then the pace will gradually pick up with new moves being added such as stepping sideways on the step, stepping down on the other side, stepping over the step with a twirl to face the other way. The whole thing is done to a strong beat – you'll find the effect a little like slow-motion morris dancing with added leotards. You may be surprised by how much you sweat. Step is one of those things where it gets easier the better you get at it. As a newbie you are putting in more effort, and getting more of a workout, than the more slick-looking steppers around you.

Enjoy high-speed cardio work with plenty of bounce but fancy something just a little more aggressive? Try a body combat class or equivalent (see IDEA 31, *Mortal combat*).

Try another idea...

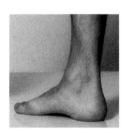

'To get fit, be fit, and stay fit, one had to be consistent, yet consistently change.'
GIN MILLER, step priestess

Defining idea...

How did it go?

Q **I like the idea, but I'm finding it so physically tough that I lose track of the moves just as everyone else is getting into their stride. How can I keep up?**

A *One thing at a time. First off, concentrate on the moves so you no longer worry about them, only later should you increase the difficulty level. While a 15 cm (6 inch) step is usually seen as about right for beginners, you may benefit from dropping the step to 10 cm (4 inches) (or less – just use the step platform and no supports) until you are comfortable with the routines.*

Q **I've picked this up so fast you wouldn't believe it and I can do the moves in my sleep even in the advanced class. If I want to make it tougher on myself can I increase the step height?**

A *Yes, but beyond a certain point you are risking trouble – it's reckoned that each 5 cm (2 inch) increase in height ups the difficulty level by 10 per cent. Twenty-five centimetres (10 inches) is the recommended maximum. The bottom line is that if your knee is flexing at a sharper angle than 90 degrees as you step up, you might end up damaging the joint.*

Q **I've heard that you can use hand weights to increase the difficulty in step work. What are the benefits of this?**

A *Some instructors like to introduce hand weights, which can increase muscular endurance at slow tempos. But if the class isn't designed for weights, then don't do it – you're simply increasing the risk of injury. Weights can add muscular endurance, and some people enjoy the feeling of working the upper body more, but weights won't build strength and may leave you feeling noticeably more tired with little to show for it.*

30

Hard core – core training

Why would you get in line to play with a wobble board with springs? Because you can tone your tum, boost your balance and avoid getting crocked at that forthcoming sporting challenge, that's why.

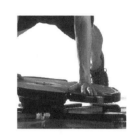

The core board is a development of the old wobble board — a board with half a football stuck on the bottom.

By adding springs the core board gives you the instability of the wobble board, but also fights back by trying to return itself to where it wants to be just as you are trying to get it to go somewhere else. The result is a heroic and dynamic struggle between man and inanimate object with the result that you get to build up the stabilising and balancing muscles of your torso. And fall off from time to time, naturally.

Core boards have a major advantage over Swiss balls or wobble balls. If you try to rotate your body in a vertical axis the core board will try to push you back the other way. To combat that you have to use muscular force to counter the turning action as well as keep your balance. It makes for a varied and active workout but is still quite gentle – the core board was created by the physical therapist to Canada's national soccer team to help rehabilitate injured football players. OK, OK, so none of us can name a single Canadian football player, but on the other hand you've never heard of any of them staying injured either, right?

Here's an idea for you... **Getting particularly confident on the basic balances? OK, just for a moment try shutting your eyes as you do them. It should throw you off enough to make it interesting without sending you careering across the studio.**

The idea now is that not only does the board help build up core strength by recruiting as many muscles as possible to help balance, it also reduces your risk of getting crocked at that company five-a-side/netball tournament. By gently 'surprising' your muscles with its twists and turns it strengthens them and makes them much less likely to be shocked or injured when you make that desperate lunge to get away from that nippy young defender from Bought Ledger.

Plus it's fun. It's really fun – giggle-out-loud sort of fun, and when was the last time you did that in an abs class?

Try another idea... **Enjoy putting your body off-balance and toning that lower torso? Course you do, which is why you should take a look at IDEAS 11 and 12 on balls and learn to love the big round world of rainbow-coloured vinyl.**

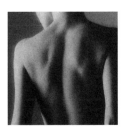

WHAT CAN I EXPECT?

You'll start off with some stretches to loosen the hamstrings, hip flexors and calves, then a few simple balances on the board. Next you'll move on to a little bit of rhythmic movement (don't worry, there's nothing you could call choreography here) interrupted with stationary balances. Expect to spend a fair amount of time on the end of the board with one leg in the air doing squats and delivering slow motion (and very wobbly) kicks sideways, forwards and backwards. Imagine a Bruce Lee film acted out by Grandpa Simpson.

After lateral balances and forward balances you'll move on to a bit of upper body and obliques work, possibly kneeling on the floor with one arm balanced on the board and twisting away for all you're worth.
It sounds silly, it looks silly…it feels great.

'With all the benefits that Reebok Core Training offers, plus the fun, high-energy total body workout the Core Board provides, we're excited to delight the world again with an innovative, unprecedented program that we believe is the future of athletic and strength conditioning.'
KATHY O'CONNELL, Reebok executive, getting very excited over what is, after all, a spring sandwiched between two boards.

Defining idea…

Q   **I fell off.**

A   *You too huh? It happens. If you're anything like me it happens a lot. Get used to it and get back on.*

Q   **I've been doing this for a while but I'm still nothing like as stable as most of the people around me. Will I ever get better?**

A   *Certainly. While it's true that some people are naturally better at balance, most of us have learnt (or forgotten) it as we go along. If you don't do much physical movement or you always do the same movement you will take longer to learn how to stabilise. Console yourself with the thought that if you are finding it harder, then your muscles are getting a more thorough workout than those poised people around you.*

Q   **Simply put, whenever I'm trying to balance on one leg I fall over. That can't be right, can it?**

A   *Are you locking your knee and trying to balance on a straight leg? It's a common mistake because it feels like it would be more stable, but it isn't. Make sure your weight-bearing leg is slightly bent at the knee as it will be more flexible and more likely to adapt to the shifting weight of your body on the board.*

134

31

Mortal combat – BodyCombat and co.

Mixing martial arts moves and music is a trend sweeping gyms world-wide. Work off some aggression along with the pounds.

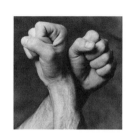

Skipping around beating the hell out of thin air might not sound like an appropriate pastime for a grown adult but it's a rare gym these days that doesn't feature body combat, tae box or another exotically named equivalent.

Perhaps they're a sign of these stressful times, a tribute to the subtle artistry of Jean Claude Van Damme and co. or therapy for work/lovelife hassles. Whatever. The fact is that for a lot of people aggressive workouts work.

BodyCombat is the trademark name of the workout from the Les Mills company (the guys who brought you BodyPump) and if your gym isn't a subscriber then it's like as not have another flavour with a different name but much the same moves. The moves themselves are taken from boxing, tai chi, kickboxing and tae kwondo, choreographed into pumping, all-dancing all-kicking extravaganzas. As well as delivering a great cardio workout and blowing off steam, they are often trumpeted as 'empowering' or 'confidence-building' – but don't get carried away and try to quell pub fights with your fabulous air kicks.

Here's an idea for you...

While most of the martial-arts-moves-to-music are essentially the same, there is one thing that separates the men from the boys/women from the girls. That is the element of contact. Ask at your gym if any of the courses with martial arts moves actually involve contact pads, then trot along and try it. With contact versions of martial arts workouts you still warm up by heaving punches and launching kicks at the atmosphere, but you then move on to trying to land them on someone. This isn't as painful as it sounds. You'll be divided up into pairs and one of you holds the pad while the other launches attacks on it. Padded gloves protect the puncher's pandies. Hand pads can be held horizontally for you to deliver uppercuts to, or vertically to practice jabs. Full body pads can be held up to act as targets for kicks or hooks. You'll get to take turns at holding or hitting the pads. Holding the pads can be more of a workout than you'd expect. I remember one partner who purposefully strapped on the gloves and informed me that she'd thrown her boyfriend out the day before. I spent the next half an hour being driven backwards by shuddering blows while praying that the protective pad didn't give up the ghost.

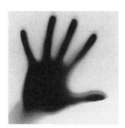

Mortal arts certainly beat the stuffing out of old-style aerobic classes but be aware that even though they are billed as non-contact that doesn't mean they are no-impact for your body. The bouncing up and down, sudden changes of direction and shooting your limbs out in various directions are all exhilarating but hard on the joints. You'll need to be in fairly good shape, and wearing shoes with good ankle support.

If explosive bursts of power are your thing, then work on your strength with plyometric exercises – see IDEA 22, *Explode into action.*

Try another idea...

'If you always put a limit on everything you do, physical, or anything else it will spread into your work and into your life. There are no limits. There are only plateaus, and you must not stay there, you must go beyond them.'
BRUCE LEE, finding time for philosophy in between clouting bad guys.

Defining idea...

Q   I love it but I'm too exhausted to finish the class. What can I do to make it through to the bitter end?

How did it go?

A   *Martial arts moves like these are hard on the body because they require both a level of simple endurance to keep going for an hour but also recruit the 'fast twitch' muscles needed for explosive movements. To get better you will need to work on cardio endurance (try the treadmill – IDEA 9) and also plyometric power (IDEA 22, Explode into action).*

Q **Front kicks make sense, but when I try a side kick my leg sort of flops out sideways like the reaction you get when the doctor tests your reflexes. All the others look like they could kick down walls. What am I doing wrong?**

A *Side kicks may not come so naturally but don't let that put you off. Turn your hips and your shoulders away from the target so you are side on and, without twisting your torso, turn your neck to look over your shoulder at the place you want to kick. Then raise your front knee up to hip height, keeping your heel close to your body so your bent leg is tensed like a spring. Aim low (knee) for beginners, don't raise your sights to the groin until you are more experienced. Keep your abs tight as you fire out the kick with the edge of the foot forward to strike the surface. Don't think of kicking the target, imagine kicking right through the target. Bring the leg back to that loaded spring position before setting it back on the ground.*

Q **I'm enjoying the contact martial arts class at my gym but when my partner lands a punch on the pads it rattles my fillings and when it's my turn she laughs at my feebleness. Any ideas?**

A *Don't try and throw a punch using just the strength in your arms. A really forceful punch means putting your whole body behind it. As you punch you should twist at the waist and put your shoulder behind the arm. Getting your whole upper body in on the act also makes for a better workout. As with good kicking don't aim to hit the target, aim to drive right through it.*

32

Eating and Drinking

It may well be all the eating and drinking that has led you to the gym but now is not the time to stop. The trick is to know what to eat and drink before, during and after training.

Since weight loss is a major driving force in gym city, it's a fair bet that if you're going to the gym you're probably also watching what you eat.

Fair enough, but if you're trying to starve yourself and sweat your little cotton socks to a pulp all at the same time, then you're on a highway to fatigue, grumpiness and burn out. Yes we all want to burn off our fat reserves, and putting more fuel in as we exercise may seem counterintuitive, but if you want to get the most out of your gym sessions you should learn to snack for success.

The following recommendations are aimed at those doing cardio/calorie-burning exercises. The standard wisdom in the body-building world is that you can burn fat, or you can build muscle, but trying to do both at once is counterproductive. You're better off burning fat first before moving on to muscling up.

BEFORE

If you head for the gym first thing before work, then the usual recommendation is a light breakfast based on carbohydrates (like cereals). Breakfast bars and sports bars

139

Your gym may have drinking fountains but they won't help you keep an eye on how much you drink. Make sure you take a large (three-quarters of a litre or more) drinking bottle with you to the gym and keep it to hand whenever you're in a class or on a machine. If bag space is a problem, then go to a camping shop and get a fold-flat polythene drinking pouch that you can roll up when it's empty.

can provide a good balance but be careful because a lot of breakfast bars have a very high fat content. Sports bars usually provide a balance of carbs, protein and fat, but are high calorie so snack on them all day and you might as well have eaten all the pies.

A lot of people find it hard to stomach anything before a workout which isn't a disaster (unless your workout is a three-hour run). It's probably more important to consider what you shouldn't eat, rather than what you should. Big no-nos include:

Sugar – Ignore anyone telling you that a chocolate bar is great before you play. Sure it contains loads of energy, but a lot of it is in the form of sugar. You'll get a short, sharp, sugar high followed later by a sugar low. Combine that with the natural trough that follows a hormone and adrenaline charged workout and you'll leave the gym grumpy and blue.

Protein – Yes it's the building block for making muscle but it's also a pig to digest. Take it easy on the high-protein foods before a session.

DURING

Drink! As Father Jack used to say to Father Ted. Of course he also used to roar 'Girls!' and 'Feck!' but we'll leave those till later. In the course of an hour's intense exercise you can lose a kilo of bodyweight. Sounds good, but beware: that kilo is all water and if you don't put this back into your system your cells malfunction and your blood volume decreases. So drink, but to rehydrate in a hurry you should opt for so-called isotonic sports drinks. The essential ingredients in a sports drink are 6–8 per cent carbs (usually in the form of glucose) and 'electrolytes' (usually sodium) to replace the minerals lost through sweat. Manufacturers make all sorts of claims for rival sports drinks but the key thing about isotonic drinks is that they are absorbed much faster than water because they more closely match the mineral balance of our body fluids. Incidentally this also makes them nifty for morning-after rehydration – not that a dedicated athlete like yourself would know anything about that.

Endurance athletes also favour energy gels which may be isotonic or may need to be washed down with water. These provide energy on the go but you're unlikely to be needing them unless your intensive sessions are over an hour long.

Sorted out what to put into your body? Fine, now make sure you've taken care of what to wrap yourself up in with IDEA 1, *Looking the part*.

Try another idea...

AFTER

'Never eat more than you can lift.'
MISS PIGGY

Defining idea...

Shoving food into your face immediately after exercise may seem to miss the point but it's an important time to eat. First, you want to avoid the energy trough that can follow a workout because your long-term motivation is going to be a lot better if you end up feeling great all day. Second, the body is a complex thing and if you make huge energy demands on it and then don't feed it you may be sending it the wrong messages. If your body believes times are hard with lots of work and no food it may even try to hold on to fat reserves. Reassure it that there's grub a plenty by guzzling a sports bar, a sports drink or a banana after your work-out to give it some easily digested carbs to get going on.

How did
it go?

Q I exercise in the morning and only have a light breakfast. How come I still feel like I have a cannonball sat in my stomach?

A   *Could be you're taking in too much protein. Some people are especially sensitive and even milk may cause a problem. Try swapping your cornflakes for a (low fat) cereal or sports bar and see if it makes any difference.*

Q I go to the gym to feel better and I do, well I do for about twenty minutes afterwards and then I feel tired and negative. Any ideas?

A   *Eating immediately after exercise helps even out the peak and trough effect. Some experts say the food should be eaten within fifteen minutes of the end of exercising to get the best effect. Try including a banana, a flavoured (skimmed) milk shake or a sports bar along with your gym kit and start scoffing before you shower.*

Q What about protein supplements?
A   *Bodybuilders may love them but they are trying to bulk up and too much protein can make life tough for your kidneys. Unless you're edging towards the extreme end of the fitness spectrum it's probably better to focus on getting a balanced diet than it is to worry about supplements. If in doubt see a doctor or nutritionist.*

33

Pump that body

Hanker after muscle tone but have no intention of hanging out with the grunting meatheads in the weights room? Prefer your exercise to be set to motivational music with clear instructions about what to do? That doesn't sound so unreasonable, in fact it sounds a lot like BodyPump.

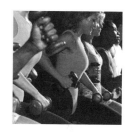

BodyPump came out of New Zealand in 1990 and has proved an instant hit in gyms worldwide because it answers an obvious need

Lots of us are looking for more toned upper bodies, and we've come to realise that cardio work and normal aerobics aren't going to do the job. There have always been weights of course, but the macho atmosphere of the weights room can be a serious turn off and the complexity of the equipment can be offputting. Cue BodyPump (a patent of the frighteningly successful Les Mills company) and its imitators.

By combining barbells and bench (in the form of an aerobics step) the BodyPump routine is designed to give a complete body workout. On the way it gives you an idea of all the most common weights moves – squats, lunges, bench press, shoulder press, curls, etc. It also follows good form in the order of working. First there's a warm-up, then the big muscle groups and combinations are worked with squats, bench press and back work. Then it moves on to focus on smaller muscles like biceps and triceps, the shoulders and finally the abs and a cool-down and stretch.

It's pretty much a lesson in good workout procedure. By using light weights (which the user chooses) and high repetitions the aim is very much on toning, not on building muscle. It won't turn you into Arnie. Bodybuilders despise it partly for this very reason. Non-bodybuilders just give thanks.

Here's an idea for you...

The squat is often a problem area in pump for those worried about their back. Your back should never arch when bearing the weight and the way to ensure that is to thrust your buttocks out as you descend. Some find that easier than others, however, so there are some variations if you're having trouble and worrying about your back:

FRONT SQUAT – Place the bar across the front of your shoulders in front of your neck. Cross your arms to give more stability on the grip. Front loading can help keep your spine neutral.

THREE-LEGGED SQUAT – Use your own bodyweight to squat with no weight plates. Stand the bar itself out in front of you vertically resting on the floor to spread your weight.

PLATE SQUAT – This works on the same principle as the front squat but take a single plate and hug it to your chest as you squat.

Look around in a pump class and you'll quickly see that a lot, probably most, of those working away are women – which is the hallmark of BodyPump's success. It's clear what to do, the basic pattern stays the same, the instructor is there to show you and the whole thing is set to thumping music to keep the blood up. Of course it appeals. Nor is it just 'weights lite' for newbies – it's a pretty good all-round workout for anyone interested in toning. Because it uses free weights and thus recruits the balancing muscles, and because it imposes the discipline of working all the main muscle groups, it's a lot more thorough than most of those hesitant sessions you see people putting in on the fixed weight machines.

BodyPump is based around many and relatively rapid repetitions with a light weight. For a completely opposite approach to building strength take a look at IDEA 25, *Take it slow.*

Try another idea...

'That which does not kill me makes me stronger.'
FREDERICH NIETZSCHE

Defining idea...

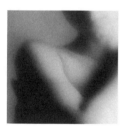

145

How did
it go?

Q   **I find I can lift a lot of weight in the squats section but the bar itself digs into my neck when it rests on my shoulders. Any ideas?**

A   *BodyPump sells a foam bar protector to help with exactly that but it's a lot cheaper to take your towel and wrap it around the bar before you hoist it to your shoulders for the squats.*

Q   **The instructor always stops me when I get tired during the bench press and drop the bar nearly to my chest. Why is it so important to keep the bar higher?**

A   *The real point is not so much the chest, it's your elbows dipping below the level of your bench. When you let the bar get that low it puts stress on the connecting tissues in the shoulder and the bench press section of BodyPump is trying to work the pec muscles of your chest.*

Q   **I can do all of the exercises without trouble except one – the lunge. Here I am always being corrected for not having my body straight. What can I do?**

A   *Most of us have trouble getting the lunge right. Try using the Smith machine (IDEA 24, Meeting Mr Smith) to do lunges – the machine forces you to move only in a vertical axis so you can focus on getting your leg position right without worrying that you're leaning forwards.*

34

In the swim I: Splash with style

Swimming is one of the best all-round exercises known, but most of us, if we're honest, are no better at swimming than we were at school. Learn to cut a dash as you splash.

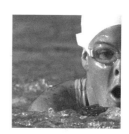

Swimming involves your whole body. It works your heart and lungs, it increases strength, flexibility and endurance, but involves very little risk of injury.

It is often picked out as one of the few exercises where even a very hard workout leaves you feeling good and ready for the rest of the day.

When you signed up for your gym a lot was made of the fact that it has a swimming pool, right? It's a big selling point for gyms, and often one of the reasons given for choosing one over another by new members all picturing themselves enjoying a refreshing dip and cutting a dashing figure as they surge up and down the lanes.

Six months later and those would-be dolphins are either forming hippo herds in the shallow end, or avoiding the pool altogether in favour of cardio machines they understand better. Unless you're one of the dedicated few fish people it can be hard

Here's an idea for you... **As you focus more on making your stroke efficient it becomes time to take up a new sport – stroke golf. Swim a length and count the number of strokes it takes you to complete it. Now using what you've learnt from swimming with arms or legs only try to swim the length using fewer strokes. See how far you can bring down your score by concentrating on getting the most progress out of the fewest number of strokes.**

to make progress in the pool. The default option is just to flounder up and down a bit the same as ever. Which is fine but limited since it doesn't lead to any improvement in style or strength. The real answer is a swimming coach, but since these aren't always an option here are some thoughts about how to examine your own swimming, and some exercises you can do to improve it. At the very least they will make a change from the end-to-end plodding.

BREAK IT DOWN

Whether your favourite stroke is front crawl, back crawl, breaststroke or butterfly it has both an arm action and a leg action. Co-ordinating both actions was one of the hurdles you had to overcome when you first learnt that stroke but now if you want to get better you're going to have to get uncoordinated, just for the moment. Swimming is a fairly complex set of movements and rhythms and it sometimes helps to break them down in order to focus on individual elements. Here we're going to focus on just the arm, and then just the leg movements in isolation.

FLOATS AND PULL-BUOYS

You'll remember the humble float from your days as a learner. The pull-buoy may be less familiar but basically it's just a float that's shaped so it's easier to hold between your legs. If your pool doesn't have any pull-buoys a normal float will do – it'll just try harder to get away from you.

LEGS

Scissors kick, butterfly kick or frog leg strokes should all be enough on their own to propel you from one end of the pool to the other. Grab a float, hold it out in front of you with both hands and use only your legs to swim.

If you have a pool and you want to make the most of it, why not try your hand at triathlon – take a look at IDEA 28, *Try a tri*.

Try another idea...

ARMS

As with legs, only in reverse. Lodge a pull buoy or a float (you may need two depending on your natural buoyancy or lack of it) between your thighs. Now set off up the pool using only your arm stroke.

In both of these cases the aim is not to be fast, but to be comfortable. If you are tired after a length, then you may want to work on putting less effort into the stroke, and instead getting more out by means of better form (see *How did it go?*).

'Fitness is something that happens to you while you're practising good technique.'
TERRY LAUGHLIN, swim coach and director of the Total Immersion school of swimming

Defining idea...

How did it go?

Q   I like swimming but chlorine hurts my eyes, and goggles either leak or else they're so tight they seem to dig into my eye sockets. Any ideas?

A   Different goggles suit different face shapes so try a few different ones to find the softest. Go for a soft rim, or look out for 'mask' type goggles which look a bit like diving masks but without the nosepiece. These spread the point of contact and give you a bigger field of vision which can also reassure some swimmers.

Q   Without the help of my feet I find it hard to steer straight? Any ideas?

A   Try making it worse to make it better. Take a large rubber band and put it around your ankles. With pull buoy in place set off up the pool. Now you'll really feel it if you fishtail. Concentrate on making your legs follow your body in a perfectly straight line as it could be that you are wasting energy by jack-knifing laterally as you swim.

Q   Smoothness and technique are all very well but I also want to build up my strength. What can I do to make swimming more muscular?

A   Have you tried paddles? No kidding – paddles are to hands what fins are to feet. They consist of a plastic board that straps to your hand, making it larger. That takes more effort to pull back through the water and so works your shoulders and laterals more. Most good sports shops sell them in small, large and medium sizes. But be careful: if you've never used them before, start with small or medium sizes – leaping in with large ones can strain shoulder muscles.

35

In the swim II: What a drag

Style is everything in swimming. Good style means ease, speed and the confidence to keep on going for hour after hour.

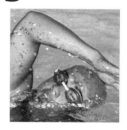

Swimming is style delimited.

That doesn't mean you're going to get banned from the pool because you swim like a shopping trolley, it just explains why trying to go faster by throwing more effort at it will simply get you nowhere. It's all down to drag. The faster you move through water the greater the drag created by your body displacing the water as you go (water is twelve times more resistant than air). Which means that there's a limit to how much faster you can go by swimming harder. Unless you do something about that drag factor the muscle you throw at the stroke will be cancelled out by the extra drag you create. Remember that and scoff the next time you see some Neanderthal thinking he's impressing everyone by thrashing his way up the pool. The answer is to learn to streamline your body and reduce the drag so as to swim smarter, not harder.

Think about your body posture in the water and try to swim more like a fish and less like a labrador. That means no more looking forwards (which presents your face to the water) but instead looking down and trying to make your whole body like a spear, with your head and spine in line.

The other area where our posture often works against us is that we allow our hips to sink into the water. Thanks to our lungs our chest cavities are a buoyant flotation

Total Immersion is the coaching philosophy of Terry Laughlin who has set up an entire business around the principle that the key to good swimming is to make yourself more streamlined, rather than hammering up and down for hours at a time. Total immersion classes tend to be a bit pricey but if they come to your gym they may be worth it and the approach has had a lot of success with adult swimmers. If the classes are too costly there is also a book and video of the same name.

aid stuck between our shoulders. In order to position our whole bodies higher in the water (so reducing drag) the best approach is to try and push the chest, rather than the hips, into the water so that the buoyancy forces us up.

Although most of us see swimming as something you do on your front or your back, we are actually most streamlined when tilted onto our sides and that's how we should swim front crawl. Instead of keeping your body flat in the water and turning your head right round to breathe at every stroke, try rolling your entire torso with the stroke. You should turn sideways with your pulling arm going deep and your head barely needing to turn at all to clear the water and suck in the air. It's a great technique for those who get neck ache from turning their heads so high to get their mouths out of the water.

Try a stroke drill called catch-up to concentrate on your front crawl arm stroke. The idea is to perfect the long, streamlined swimming position that helps fishboys and fishgirls glide their way from one end of the pool to the other. In the normal stroke the forward arm is pulling back as the recovering arm prepares to enter the water. In this drill one arm stays stretched out in front of you as the other arm completes the pull back part of the stroke. As that arm enters the water you slide it forward so both of your arms are now momentarily outstretched in front of you and only then start to pull back with the other arm. Focus on trying to make yourself longer in the water.

Instead of trying to avoid water resistance, how about revelling in it and using it to develop your strength? Try IDEA 42, *Aqua aerobics and water running*, to find out how.

Try another idea...

'The man who is swimming against the stream knows the strength of it.'
WOODROW WILSON

Defining idea...

153

How did it go?

Q   I've heard of swimmers using beepers. What are they?

A   *Beepers set a rhythm just as a metronome does for a musician. By timing hand entry into the water on each stroke to the beep from the pacer, swimmers pace themselves to complete a certain number of strokes per distance.*

Q   Are there swimming fins for swimmers, rather than divers/snorkellers?

A   *Yes, look out for Zoomers, or Hydro Training Finz which are softer and smaller than the large fins used for scuba. If you want something a bit usual and find normal fins uncomfortable, look out for Tritan fins which are virtually round.*

Q   I'm trying to get from one end of the pool to the other using just my front crawl leg stroke (see IDEA 34, *In the swim I*). How come I'm being passed by kids with waterwings?

A   *Take the opportunity of pushing that float in front of you to pop your head up so your ears are clear of the water. Now listen to yourself. Can you hear your feet splashing or churning the water? Any splash means that they are wasting energy thrashing the surface of the water.*

36

Piling on the Pilates

The ballerinas' secret for long and lean muscles is now recognised as having benefits for everyone from recovering rugby players to recovering couch potatoes. You don't have to don a tutu to get the most from these midsection moves.

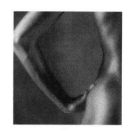

Joseph H. Pilates was no ballerina.

A puny youth who suffered from rickets, asthma and rheumatic fever, he developed his now famous technique in a concerted attempt to overcome his own physical weaknesses. He didn't have the resources of a modern gym to help him either. He mainly worked up his theories when banged up in an internment camp during World War I. What he did have was time, a fairly confined amount of space and minimal equipment (apart from bedsprings, but we won't deal with that here). Despite, or perhaps because of that, our Joseph forged himself a new body, and in the process a career as gymnast, boxer, circus performer and eventually physical educator.

His theories have been taken up and moved on by generations of practitioners, but certain characteristics and the basic principles remain unchanged. Without going through them all, the keys are concentration, precise control of movement, an understanding of the role and technique of breathing, and of the importance of building a strong physical core to anchor all other movements and exercise.

Here's an idea for you...

Joseph H. was born too soon to know the full joy of bouncy vinyl Swiss balls but plenty of Pilates practitioners since then have seized on the Swiss ball as an exercise tool. Doing Pilates on a ball gives you the opportunity to stretch further than before while still being comfortably supported. It's also oddly soothing. Give it a go.

WHAT CAN I EXPECT?

You'll start with mat work and perhaps a large sausage of plastic foam. Initially a lot of work will focus on making you aware of specific parts of your body and in particular the muscles of your stomach and the bones that you sit on. Next come simple movements such as rolling up into a sitting position or lifting legs and shoulder blades off the deck. These help you realise how different parts of the body work together – for example how lying on your front and pulling your shoulder blades down should lift your chest slightly off the ground. The moves are all done slowly, with considerable emphasis on breathing correctly, and repetitions are very few in number. If that sounds a bit cushy, then think again. The degree of concentration, plus the effort of tensing muscles in unfamiliar ways, makes for surprisingly hard work. You would have to be some kind of twisted genius to injure yourself during a Pilates session, however, so it suits all ages and levels of physical strength and flexibility. It also promotes a general feeling of well-being due to measured breathing, gentle pace and the sense of muscle control. That control is also the key to why it appeals so much to recovering athletes. If that's what draws you, then make sure you signal your injury to the instructor before launching into a class.

Among the benefits of Pilates are a greater attention to the deeper-lying muscles of the core, such as the transversus which lies under the abs. For athletes, this core strength approach gives greater balance and power. Dancers appreciate the suppleness encouraged by moves, and there are those who swear that it improves posture so much that you can end up taller!

If core strength is what you're after, then try the core training classes covered in IDEA 30, *Hard core*. Or if you're working on your own, take a look at the exercises using the Swiss ball in IDEAS 11 and 12.

Try another idea...

'Physical fitness is the first requisite of happiness. Our interpretation of physical fitness is the attainment and maintenance of a uniformly developed body with a sound mind fully capable of naturally, easily, and satisfactorily performing our many and varied daily tasks with spontaneous zest and pleasure.'
JOSEPH H. PILATES

Defining idea...

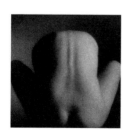

157

How did
it go?

Q   **Why is there so much emphasis on 'rolling' up rather than sitting up?**

A   *As the man himself once said, 'in coming up and going down, roll your spine like a wheel. Vertebra by vertebra try to roll and unroll.' Don't be confused by the grammar, the point is to try and feel the different parts of your body and understand the way they move together even in supposedly simple actions.*

Q   **The instructor tells me to breathe out. I breathe out, and still they stare at me. Why?**

A   *In some moves in Pilates you don't just exhale, you aim to completely empty the lungs – usually so you can feel how you then fill them again using your stomach. Joseph H. himself described this as like wringing all the water out of a wet towel. Go on, wring yourself right out.*

Q   **Not sure I fully understand this neutral position when I'm lying flat on my back. I'm squeezing my stomach in as hard as possible but the instructor keeps correcting me.**

A   *Because Pilates makes us so much more aware of the stomach muscles there is a tendency to tense them and try to suck them into your spine. In the neutral position, however, this tensing of the stomach fights the natural curvature of the spine. The tip of your coccyx (tail-bone) should press down into the mat, and that should mean that a patch in the small of your back lifts up off it.*

37
The cardio cocktail
– interval training

You've probably heard of exercises being either aerobic or anaerobic...but they can be both. Blend the two together and you get a cardio cocktail that burns calories and can help push you through an exercise plateau.

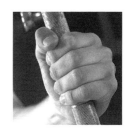

Exercise that encourages heart and lungs to work harder and get stronger is known in gym-speak as cardio(vascular), but all such exercise can also be described as aerobic.

Aerobic exercise is all about getting air into the body and getting the oxygen from it pumped around as efficiently as possible. Anaerobic exercise is the stuff that happens so fast, so intensely, that the body can't supply the oxygen needed and your muscles have to do without. Anaerobic exercise is all about short sharp shocks. Intense bursts of sprinting are anaerobic, gentle jogging is aerobic. Left to our own devices in the gym most of us settle into aerobic workout after aerobic workout.

Aerobic exercise is a great fat burner. Anaerobic exercise pushes your muscles harder, though only for short periods of time not least because it produces a by-product, lactic acid, which leaves you tired and uncomfortable. One of the best

Here's an idea for you...

If you're using a machine that has settings for different workouts, then look for one that regularly raises and decreases the resistance (probably called a 'hill-climb'). Instead of slowing down as the machine raises the resistance, set yourself a goal of a certain speed, or r.p.m. figure to maintain during those tough times. Then treat the lower resistance intervals as rests.

ways of getting rid of lactic acid is gentle aerobic exercise – what's called active recovery – which is why cool-downs are so important. Mix aerobic and anaerobic and you have a number of benefits:

■ Your normal workout becomes more challenging for your muscles promoting strength.

■ You get a more intense workout out of a shorter period of time than you would do just working away steadily.

■ It makes a change from a routine – whatever your preferred cardio exercise.

■ It can help give you that little bit of extra push to get through a performance plateau.

■ There is evidence that anaerobic exercise increases HGH (human growth hormone) levels, and HGH has anti-ageing properties.

SO WHAT DO I DO?

Pick a cardio machine, any machine. Now start off with a nice easy pace and if you or your chosen machine happen to be sporting a heart monitor (for more see IDEA 4, *Listen to your love muscle*) try and keep your heart rate at a nice gentle 55–70 per cent of your maximum. After a good 10 minutes of warm-up you're ready to up the level to 70–85 per cent of your maximum heart rate. This is the optimum for developing cardio efficiency. Five minutes of that and you can go for it with an anaerobic sprint. This means taking it up to a level of effort so intense that 20 seconds is enough to wipe you out. It's up to you to define intensive, by the way. By the end of it you should feel that your performance is dropping off as your muscles simply can't keep contracting at that intensity any longer. At which point you drop back to your nice easy level for 5 minutes of active recovery which gives you time for your heart rate to drop (see IDEA 4, *Listen to your love muscle*), and for your body to eliminate the lactic acid. This is the one time that the phrase 'going for the burn' has some meaning because in true anaerobic exercise the build-up of lactic acid causes that burning in your muscles. When you feel the burn it's time to slow down.

Fancy yourself as a bit of a runner and want to see how interval training can make you faster? Then learn about Yasso 800s in IDEA 10, *Run like Radcliffe II*.

Try another idea...

'Exercise is for people who can't handle drugs and alcohol.'
LILY TOMLIN

Defining idea...

161

How did it go?

Q   **There's no way I can do anything fast enough to feel a burn. As for 20 seconds wiping me out, I find that 20 seconds of warm-up wipes me out. Any ideas?**

A   *If your body isn't ready for it, then there's no point pushing it. Try to find a level of work that's hard for you but which you can do for a minute, then alternate one minute really hard with four minutes taking it easy. After a month or so see if you can up the intensity of that 'hard' period by increasing your speed but shortening the time you do it for.*

Q   **I'm doing this three times a week and feeling tired and demotivated. Am I overdoing it?**

A   *Could be. As a beginner try to throw in just one session a week alongside your normal workouts. As you get more confident you can up the frequency but if your workouts just leave you tired all the time then consider easing off a little.*

Q   **I only have 20 minutes free to spare in the gym. Is it worth it?**

A   *Yes. While government guidelines mention 30 minute sessions, a 20 minute session with your heartbeat raised above normal is enough to bring benefits – especially if you combine it with anaerobic intervals as above.*

38

Timesaving tips

Too pressed for time to have time for presses? Try a few of these tips to maximise those fleeting moments in the gym.

Modern life is hectic, no one has enough time, there are a gazillion things demanding your attention and since fitness isn't your profession or your first love it's the gym time that ends up suffering.

This is only natural. We're all forever promising ourselves that we'll do an extra long session next time just as soon as we've finished with this budget/school holiday/international arms deal. Little and often, however, is a much better way to exercise than sporadic blitzing. For a start it means you're less likely to half-cripple yourself by launching an under-prepared body into an overambitious workout. It's also easier mentally to keep up the momentum and the feel-good factor, not least since mega sessions with long gaps in between quickly become daunting and may lead eventually to cancelled gym memberships. Little and often makes it easier to monitor progress – a motivational bonus – plus frequent short spells in the gym will do more to raise your metabolism on a daily basis than a once-a-fortnight gut-wrenching osteopath special.

So how can you make sure you get a decent workout when you only have a few precious minutes to dedicate to the temple of toning?

We spend half our time in the weights room waiting for someone else to get off the machine we want. Meanwhile there's a rack of dumbbells sitting unused in front of a mirror somewhere. Learn the range of dumbbell exercises (see IDEA 39, *Getting smart with dumbbells I*) and you'll be able to get a whole upper-body workout without moving from the spot, or doing the gym 'excuse-me' mamba around the machines.

Try the following:

HAVE YOUR KIT READY, PACKED UP, AND BY THE DOOR

Einstein used to line up seven sets of clothes on the hangers each week so he never wasted precious brainpower deciding what to wear or trying to find it. Take his lead. When you pull stuff out of the dryer, match it up into complete sets of kit, then make sure you have a gym bag ready to go for every day. Leave it sitting by the door like a patient dog hoping to go walkies and it will be both convenient to grab and a helpful reminder to your conscience.

PLAN YOUR WORKOUT, WORK YOUR PLAN

Nobody has enough time at the gym so who are all those people wandering around from cardio room to weights and back? Be clear in advance what your workout goals are. Don't fix on a single machine – it may be in use – but decide in advance how much cardio you're going to do or what weight session you have in mind.

TRY GOING EARLY

What? Like in the morning? Working out before the day gets its claws into you means you start out feeling good and get your metabolism up and running. There are also fewer people and it's hard not to feel virtuous which makes it more likely you'll be back for more tomorrow.

TRAIN WITH YOUR BELOVED/KIDS/MATES

Don't force fitness to compete with friendships and lovelife – it will come a sad second and if it doesn't you will become a sad individual. See if you can mix gym/social life by training with friends and family. This may mean thinking a little laterally. You may have trouble getting your spouse to show up to an abs class, for example, but swap it for something more fun like a core class (see IDEA 30, *Hard core*) and you can frolic with the whole family.

DON'T REST, CROSS-TRAIN

Your gym tells you to spend no more than 20 minutes on a machine? Fine, just leap straight off it and onto another one. Take ten on each if you like. Forty minutes working on a mix of rower/treadmill/bike will give you a more thorough workout than the same time spent plodding away at the same machine. It uses different muscles and psychologically allows you to put more effort because you know you're changing soon.

DON'T REST, SUPERSET

Normal practice if you're doing weights is to rest at least 30 seconds in between sets. Well don't. Instead switch straight to an exercise that works the opposite set of muscles and cut to and fro between the two with no rest time at all. For example, if you're working biceps, then alternate with a triceps press. Pair chest press exercises with lateral pull downs. Hamstrings with quads, etc.

Try another idea...

If time's winged chariot is not only drawing near but seeming double-parked on your shoulder then maximise your time with interval training – see IDEA 37, ***The cardio cocktail***. For strength training in half the time, check out IDEA 25, ***Take it slow***.

Defining idea...

'That's so when I forget how to spell my name, I can still find my clothes.'
STU GRIMSON, American football player, explaining why he has a photograph of himself on his locker.

165

How did it go?

Q **There's this one machine I'm in love with but I have a rival in the form of a pumped-up gorilla who sits on it doing nothing. I have to get to work on time, and can't afford to hang around. What do I do?**

A *Correct form here is to smile, look keen and ask if you can share the machine by alternating sets. The gorillas almost always agree because it gives them a chance to chortle at the difference between what you set the weight to and what they then lift.*

Q **I'd love to go to the gym every day but I'm on the road and only use hotel gyms. I can't carry around a different set of kit for every day and I don't want to smell like someone who uses the same damp kit three days in a row. Any ideas?**

A *IDEA 1, Looking the part, explains the virtues of wicking fabrics. If you have nylon shorts and a wicking top you can rinse them out in the shower afterwards and they'll be dry in a couple of hours. For a sweat towel go to a camping shop and get a small 'pack' towel which you can also rinse and dry out quickly.*

Q **The gym bag by the door is a nice idea but I'm already struggling under the weight of briefcases and computers so I rarely pick it up. Can you help?**

A *Ever thought of renting a locker at the gym? Most gyms rent lockers relatively cheaply and it means that (a) you never waste time looking for one and (b) when you open it your shoes and stuff are already there. Which means you just have to squeeze a fresh T-shirt, and a pair of shorts (plus, perhaps, a sports bra) into your briefcase.*

39

Getting smart with dumbbells I: Upper body

There's more to dumbbells than biceps curls. Combined with some simple accessories, like a bench and your body, they offer one of the simplest and most effective workouts. Plus there's never a queue for them.

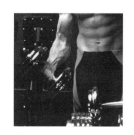

Dumbbells have a bad name from years of association with muscle-bound freaks doing endless biceps curls.

What's easily forgotten is that they offer more range of movement than any other weights apparatus (you try waving a barbell over your head with one hand) and are also great for chest, abs, legs and back. What's more I can virtually guarantee that you'll never have to queue for them. If one set of dumbbells is in use, there's bound to be another pair of a different weight that you can use for another exercise in your extensive dumbbell repertoire. You don't have a repertoire of dumbbell moves? Then read on.

All of these moves are best done in front of a mirror. Primarily this is to watch for good form but we all know that it's really so you can admire your fab new leopard-skin leotard.

Here's an idea for you... **Enjoying the weights work and want to get a bit fancy? Most of these moves can be done swapping the bench for the Swiss ball to add a little imbalance to the move and bring the core muscles of the midsection into the action. Don't be tempted to start off with overly heavy dumbbells though, as you will look a right muppet if you overbalance and fall off the ball spilling dumbbells in all directions.**

ARMS

It would be churlish not to mention the biceps curl so – just as a reminder – stand feet shoulder-width apart, don't move your shoulder, and keep the smooth control on both lift and descent. For a bit of variety try a hammer grip in which you hold the dumbbell so it's vertical in your hand at the top of the lift, as if hefting a hammer.

If you have a bench to hand, then sit on it facing the mirror and rest your right elbow on your right inner thigh just behind the knee. Now you should have completely isolated the biceps during the movement with no shoulder involvement at all.

Triceps time. Standing up, hold the dumbbell in one hand, straighten your arm above you and then gently bend your elbow so the weight comes to rest just behind your neck. Now, without moving anything but your forearm at the elbow, straighten and relax the arm to work the triceps.

Remember that bench? Great, if you have a bench then keep your left leg on the floor and put your right knee on the bench. Lean forward and grip the bench with your right arm. With the dumbbell in your left hand, pull your elbow up so your upper arm is parallel to the floor. Now extend your forearm out straight behind you and back to work those tris.

SHOULDERS

Dumbbells really are the thing when it comes to the deltoids in the shoulders. With a light weight in each hand, stand with feet shoulder-width apart and knees slightly bent and arms by sides. Now lift both arms out straight up to shoulder height. Relax and lift again but this time with arms straight up to the front so you end up in the classic 'sleepwalker' position. Repeat. Lots.

CHEST

Try the close-grip bench press – Take a dumbbell in each hand and lie on the bench. Extend both arms straight up above your chest. Lower the weights with your elbows sliding past your sides and stop before the dumbbells reach your chest itself. Repeat.

Chest fly – Using a lighter pair of dumbbells than those you used for the above exercise, lie on the bench with the weights extended straight up over your chest. Now bend your elbows slightly (and keep them bent) and lower the dumbbells out and to the sides so you're arms are out sideways like someone throwing the shutters open in the morning. Bring the dumbbells down until your upper arms are parallel to the floor – don't take it down any further as it will stress the connecting tissue in the front of your shoulders. Smoothly return to start position. Repeat.

Try another idea...

If using light free weights is appealing, but you don't intend to get in line for the weights room, perhaps you should give a pump class a try and have a total body workout to music using a barbell. Try IDEA 33, *Pump that body.* If you've enjoyed using your upper body with the dumbbells try IDEA 40, *Getting smart with dumbbells II,* to find out about working your lower body.

Defining idea...

'Big Muscles, "Six Pack" Abs, Popularity and Respect Among Men. All it takes is just 15 minutes a day.'
CHARLES ATLAS touts his wares.

BACK

Reverse fly – Effectively this is the fly move for the chest but flipped over so you're face down. Start face down on the bench with the dumbbells hanging down, then, keeping your arms lightly bent, pull your shoulder blades together and lift the arms out wide to each side. Keep the movement slow and return back to the start position. Don't let the weights drop onto the floor or be tempted to drop your arms suddenly after reaching the top of the lift.

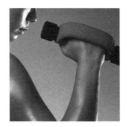

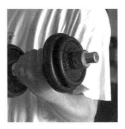

Q   I'm new to all this. How much weight should I use?

How did it go?

A   Obviously that varies from person to person but as a general rule try to pick a dumbbell that you can lift between 12 and 20 times. That's very light for strength work, but if you're a beginner you'll also need to strengthen your connective tissues and get used to the weights without risking tearing anything by trying to heave huge lumps of iron around.

Q   OK, and as I get used to, even bored with, the light weights I can start piling on the iron. Right?

A   Most people start off by finding that they can increase weight really quickly. That can be a delusion though, because it often means they're getting used to the moves and are learning to cheat by using momentum or by getting other muscles to muscle in on the act. Some experts advise no more than 10 per cent increases per week. The real test is that you shouldn't even think of upping the weight unless you're confident you can complete at least three sets of ten lifts with perfect form.

Q   Form, form, form – I'm not a racehorse. How do I know whether my form is good?

A   Swallow your pride, find an instructor and get them to supervise you through your sets. Remember that it's oh so easy to let our ego get in the way of listening to advice.

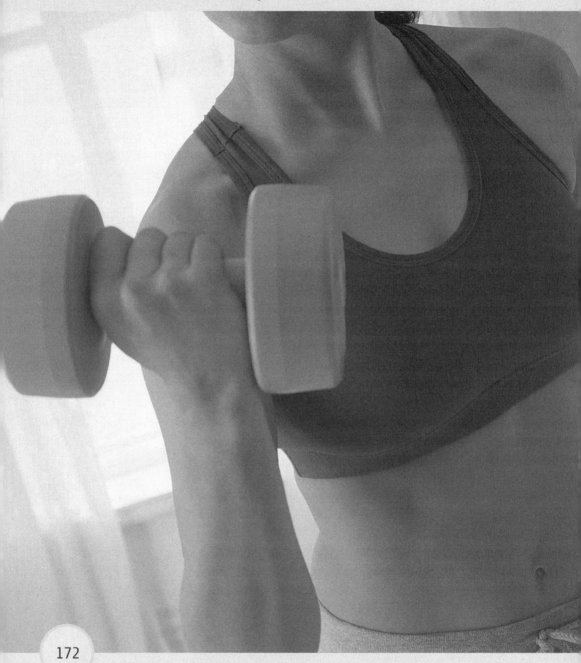

40

Getting smart with dumbbells II: Lower body

Dumbbells aren't just for arms. Here's how hand-held weights can work your thighs, hamstrings, calves and buttocks.

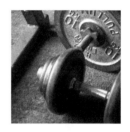

Those looking to work their lower bodies rarely give the dumbbells a thought, but you don't need huge weights to work the larger muscles, just good technique and some dumbbells.

Saunter over to the dumbbell rack, make sure you have a bench nearby and take the time to check yourself out in the mirror. By concentrating on smaller weights and better form you are about to workout and reduce your risk of injury.

SQUATS

It's not a pretty name for an exercise which should lead to leggy perfection, but it does sums up the move so precisely that it would take a good marketing team to rename it.

Start with two dumbbells (you can go fairly heavy on this one), one in each hand, at your sides, your feet shoulder-width apart, knees very slightly bent. The point of dumbbell squats is not to imitate Russian weightlifters so keep the whole movement smooth and controlled. No bouncing. No grunting.

With your shoulders pulled back, bend your knees and ease your body down as if you were slipping into a comfy chair.

Don't go so far down that either your knees move further forward, then your toes, or your bum is so low that your thighs dip down instead of being parallel to the floor. Go too low and you risk overextending and straining your muscles. Smoothly raise yourself back up to the start position.

Here's an idea for you... **Looking for a bit of variety in your lunges? Try the Bulgarian split. Drag a bench over and position it behind you. Now when you stand with your knees slightly bent and feet shoulder-width apart, stretch your rear leg out so you can rest the top of your foot on the bench behind you instead of placing it on the floor as you normally would. Now lower your body as normal into the lunge and straighten up again. Use a very light weight, or no weight at all, when you first try this as you'll feel a stretch down your quads that will make normal lunges feel like child's play.**

To hit your hip flexors try a sideways lunge. Start in the usual position but with lighter than usual weights (at least until you're used to the exercise) then take a very big step sideways as far as you can reach. Lower yourself by bending the leg that stepped out, keeping your knee moving in the same line as the foot. Smoothly straighten your knee to bring you back, and then step back to the start position.

TAKING THE LUNGE

Start as with the squat, but this time take a long step forward so your front foot is now about a yard from your back one. Keeping your torso bolt upright, lower your body by bending your legs. Your front knee shouldn't go past your toes (this is a sensible precaution for most exercises or stretches where you bend your knees). Even though you may feel a burning sensation down the length of your back leg it's the muscles of the front thigh that should be doing the work as you now lift your body back up by straightening the front leg.

For a bit of variety, and to hit the calf muscles a little more, try to switch from forward lunges, where you step forwards with one leg before lunging, and backward lunges, where you, erm, step backwards with one leg before lunging.

Try another idea...

To learn more about squats try **IDEA 49, Squat yet bijoux.** If you're worried that you can't keep your body straight during lunges, then try performing them using a Smith machine which will force you to work in a vertical axis only – see IDEA **24, Meeting Mr Smith.**

Defining idea...

Naked Guy: **'You got something against a naked body?'**

Jerry: **'I got something against yours. How about a couple deep knee bends, maybe some squat thrusts.'**
From *Seinfeld.*

How did
it go?

Q When I do lunges my knee goes way forwards beyond my toes. How do I prevent that?

A   *You need to have your front foot further forward. When you take your lunge stance you need to be much bolder in stepping further out. Even though it'll feel like it's making life harder, this is worth it to avoid strain on your knees.*

Q I try to squat or lunge down until my thigh is parallel to the floor but can't – it doesn't seem to be about using too much weight, I just don't seem to have the flexibility to make it that far. Any ideas?

A   *I'll guess you're a man. Men often have tighter hamstrings (the muscle down the back of the thigh) than women and that limits our range of movement. The best thing is to work on your hamstring stretches when your muscles are warm (see IDEA 21, At a stretch). One of the best stretches for squats is (drumroll...) squatting. Just squat down into the position as deep as is comfortable and lift yourself up afterwards by straightening your legs. Don't try to stretch when holding weights and definitely don't try and bounce yourself down into the squat position.*

Q Why do I lose my balance when I lunge?

A   *Take a look at your foot position. Having both your feet in line will make life unnecessarily hard on yourself. Instead make sure that there is a good 15 cm (6 inches) horizontal difference between the two. To get that, start your lunge with your feet side by side, then step firmly sideways with the foot that is gong to go back, before stepping backwards into position.*

41

This time it's personal – personal trainers

Personal trainers – fashion accessory for the cash-rich and time poor? Or failsafe route to fitness?

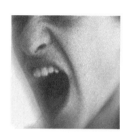

Most gyms these days offer personal training as part of their portfolio and probably promote it with all the zeal of timeshare salespeople.

At some point you will consider it, if not now, then later when you hit a motivation or performance plateau that you don't know how to get over. So what will you get for your money? And how can you decide if a personal trainer is for you?

Let's be clear about what a personal trainer means. We're not talking about having someone knock up a tailored training routine for you when you first start – all gyms should do that as a matter of course. Personal trainers will dedicate themselves to you and you alone for each hour that you book. They should assess your fitness level, set up a programme complete with goals and waypoints, and provide the motivation to achieve them.

If you're thinking of opting for personal training, ensure that the trainer:

- Has a recognised personal trainer qualification.
- Is a member of the Register of Fitness Professionals.
- Has a valid CPR (cardio-pulmonary resuscitation) certificate.

Recognised qualifications (as defined by the Register of Fitness Professionals) include:

- Future Fit Training Personal Trainer
- YMCA Personal Trainer Diploma
- Lifetime HF Personal Trainer
- FIE Certified Personal Trainer
- Premier Training Diploma
- Or a BA-level degree in sports and fitness

Here's an idea for you...

If you can't afford a personal trainer, or are a good self-starter who's just short on ideas or direction, then try an online personal trainer. They won't make tutting noises if you skip a class, but they can supply ideas and help you monitor your own progress. Try GymUser (www.gymuser.co.uk), HandBag (www.handbag.com), or the likes of www.onlinepersonaltrainer.co.uk

WHY WOULD YOU PAY THE EXTRA?

Given what you're already forking out for the gym, why would you pay extra for a personal trainer? If you have a clear idea of your fitness targets, the knowledge of how to hit them and a high level of self-motivation, then the honest answer is that you don't need a trainer. If, however, you find that motivation is a big problem, or you have an unusual target (say a new sport), or you're going nowhere and don't know what to try, then a personal trainer could be exactly what the doctor ordered.

WHAT CAN I EXPECT?

Depends entirely on what your agreed goals are. If your aim is to lose weight and tone up, then you can expect to start off with a cardio warm-up before going onto weights and moves that you wouldn't normally do. In the process you will learn a lot about form, posture, technique and the use of different pieces of equipment. It also makes the gym session an appointment, a commitment that you can't back out of, and introduces the trainer as a kind of external conscience nagging you if you let things slip. Sort of like Jiminy Cricket in tracksuit bottoms.

Prefer the pressure of someone else bullying you into shape? Then take it to its logical conclusion and sign up for a slavercise session. Take a look at IDEA 43, *Walk on the wild side.*

Try another idea...

'We do not quite forgive a giver. The hand that feeds us is in some danger of being bitten [or roundly cursed in the case of personal trainers].'
RALPH WALDO EMERSON.

Defining idea...

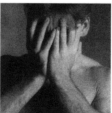

How did it go?

Q **I'm paying thirty quid an hour to be bullied and all it does is up my stress level. Any ideas?**

A *Yes, if you don't like the approach of one trainer, just try another. No two trainers will have exactly the same 'bedside manner' and you may respond much better to another one. This should be a partnership, not a marriage from hell.*

Q **My gym doesn't have a personal trainer scheme. Where can I go to find a trainer in my area?**

A *Try THEFITMAP at www.thefitmap.com which has a personal trainer finder, or the Exercise Register at www.exerciseregister.com.*

Q **My personal trainer is pushing for three sessions a week? This seems a lot. Is he just after my money?**

A *If your sessions with your personal trainer are all you do, then it's not so much, but it is an expensive way of working out. Try a compromise where you see your trainer once or twice a week and ask for them to draw up a precise plan for one or two unsupervised sessions. If the trainer isn't happy to do this, then be firm and ask why.*

42

Aqua aerobics and water running

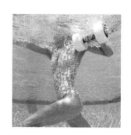

Exercising in water takes twelve times more energy than moving in air. But water supports your body and makes impact all but impossible. The result? Strength training without strain.

If your gym has a pool, then it almost certainly has a class called aqua gym or aqua aerobics.

From time to time these classes take over the pool in an odd ritual that looks like a cross between synchronised swimming and the D-Day landings with serious splashing and limbs all over the shop. If you're keen eyed you may have spotted that there are older people and pregnant women among those taking part. That's because as well as being fitness fun the wonder of aquatic exercise is that the buoyancy reduces the weight-bearing stress on your joints. It's ideal for everyone from arthritis sufferers to marathon runners suffering from overuse injuries. Heart rates are lower than equivalent land-based activities, but strength gains tend to be higher due to the constant fight against water resistance.

Because of the lower heart rate, the weightlessness and the fact that the water pressure is thought to help the return flow of blood to the heart, aqua aerobics is often recommended to the elderly. This seems to have been understood by the rest of the population as meaning that it's some kind of soft option, suited only to those

If you fancy trying water running you don't have to have a deep end and a flotation device to hand. If you can get a moment when the pool isn't packed, try walking or running up and down the lanes of the pool to get a feel for the resistance. If you can 'run' in water up to your thighs, then so much the better – try to concentrate on lifting your knees high with every step. You'll use around double the calories to run or walk for the same time you would on dry land.

who can't (or don't want to) face a real workout. This is simply wrong. Water work is a great workout for endurance, strength and flexibility – it's not because it doesn't hurt that it isn't good for you.

WHAT CAN I EXPECT?

A friendly, relaxed atmosphere for a start. Basic moves of walking, jumping sometimes with the addition of water 'weights' or 'dumbbells'. The difference between water weights and land weights is that the water versions are made of foam so that they're buoyant – the effort comes from stopping them rising rather than lifting them up.

RUNNING WATER OR WATER RUNNING?

The only group of 'serious' male athletes that have cottoned on to this are runners for whom water running is now an established technique. Water running requires a flotation device to keep you upright in the water. Other than that you try to 'run' normally but it's exhausting and works your upper body much more than traditional running.

One word of advice whether you are water running or taking part in an aqua aerobics session. Just because you are in water don't think that you won't dehydrate. These exercises are deceptive: you don't think you're doing calorie-burning exercise because it feels so gentle, and you have no idea that you are working up a sweat because you're in a pool. Make sure you take a water bottle to your pool workout.

If working out in water is to your taste, then try the swimming drills referred to in **IDEA 34, *In the swim I.***

Try another idea...

'Water, water everywhere. Nor any drop to drink.'
SAMUEL TAYLOR COLERIDGE, just to ram home the need to take a water bottle with you to the pool.

Defining idea...

183

How did
it go?

Q   How should my posture be in the pool?

A   *It's almost too easy to be comfortable in the pool – to the point where we forget about good posture, but in order to keep the spine in a good line you should aim to have your ears above your shoulders, your shoulders above your hips, with your chest out, shoulders back and your abdominals contracted.*

Q   I can see that some people aim to exercise in the deep end. Are there any benefits to that?

A   *Yes. As well as the increased calorie burn of treading water all the time it provides a workout for the core stability muscles because of the need to keep in position and counteract turning forces from the exercises themselves.*

Q   I'm enjoying the difference with aqua aerobics but is there anything I can do to maximise the effects?

A   *Aside from working in the deep end where possible, the best benefits are to be had when working in water up to your neck. Water is nearly a thousand times as dense as air and so even simple arm movements require a lot more strength (and calories burnt) if they take place entirely under the surface. If you are working out in water because of injury or joint problems, bear in mind that in shallower water you may still be bearing 50–75 per cent of your total weight. The deeper the water, the smaller that figure becomes.*

43

Walk on the wild side – pole dancing, belly dancing, s&m

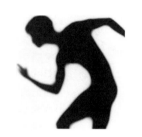

The good workout is the one you keep coming back for... and that means keeping the fun factor high.

Some people are oddly immune to the seductive charms of the exercise bike and treadmill.

They crave something a little more challenging, exciting and above all fun. Gyms are increasingly offering a range of classes that emphasis the play value alongside the carb-burning.

BELLY DANCING

All the sensual mystique of the East served up in gyms from Peckham to Pontefract. As an exercise belly dancing is a relatively gentle, low-impact aerobic session with a great deal of emphasis on hip movements which help tone midsections and in particular the obliques. 'Much more of a workout than I thought it would be' was the comment of my researcher. 'It works the stomach, hips and back. In particular it helps you get in touch with the different parts of the body especially separating out the movements of your upper and lower body since the upper body is nearly still while the hips are moving.'

Here's an idea for you...

If your gym doesn't go in for anything more exotic than an abs class, then maybe think about joining classes outside the gym or trying a session/day membership at another gym. Some gyms, such as GymBox (www.gymbox.co.uk) specialise in the more fun or off-beat activities (such as Boob Aerobics) while specialists such as Circus Space (www.thecircusspace.co.uk) focus on performing arts skills.

POLE DANCING

Pole dancing is erotic dancing using a small stage and a vertical pole that runs from floor to ceiling. You've seen it before because every US TV cop show has a scene in a pole-dancing club. As a workout it's the answer to those who love dance-based exercise but worry about upper-body strength. Because the pole moves largely involve grabbing the pole and swinging around it, there's a lot of emphasis on arm and oblique strength. More advanced moves, like swinging upside down and holding the pose, work wonders for core strength and abs. Jennifer Aniston and Angelina Jolie are said to be practitioners, though it's hard to say for sure whether that's based on reported fact or wishful thinking. Back in Blighty even Sport England is backing the pole-dancing phenomena: 'As long as it is safe, we are enthusiastic about new ways of getting people off the sofa,' commented Sport England's Chief Executive.

I'm told the atmosphere is a riot. Watch out for friction burns in unlikely places.

TRAPEZE

This one, I'm reliably informed, kicked off when *Sex and the City*'s Carrie tried out trapeze work. Trapeze involves a tough upper-body workout but also a great deal of flexibility and stabilising work. The experts at Circus Space in London also swear that it leads to great posture. Mainly, though, it's a buzz for anyone who's ever dreamt of flying through the air with the greatest of ease.

SLAVERCISE

'Mistress Victoria is like Jane Fonda, Catwoman and the hot high school gym teacher we all had a crush on, all rolled into one – with a whip!'
Slightly breathless Slavercise fan

It had to happen really. Following on from the boot camp phenomenon where sergeant major wannabes shout insults at you, a US dominatrix has marketed an alternative way to raise your blood pressure as you perform. Get ready to workout, worm. Not as yet a regular in UK gyms.

KANGOO JUMPING

When I was a kid the cartoons would regularly feature some character who ended up with springs attached to their feet and the (often unintentional) ability to bounce over tall buildings. If you ever wanted to be that character, then kangoo jumping is for you. The Kangoo boots feature a spring (leaf, rather than coil for the exercise engineers among you) on the sole which gives a bounce to the step. The class is a warm-up followed by aerobic moves with added boing. Currently the preserve of the more self-consciously groovy gyms.

If your gym doesn't stretch to such exotica but you like the idea of exercise that's for the sake of fun first and foremost, then try salsa (see IDEA 44, *Shimmy yourself svelte*) or even the core board (see IDEA 30, *Hard core*).

Try another idea...

'All life is an experiment. The more experiments you make the better.'
RALPH WALDO EMERSON

Defining idea...

Q   I asked about pole dancing down at the gym and they looked at me funny. Where can I find out more?

A   There are a number of outfits around the country but try Polestars (www.polestars.com).

Q   I'm thinking of shaking my stuff in the belly-dancing class. Any clothing tips?

A   Dedicated research comes back with the answer that any loose clothing is OK but 'psychologically you feel more in touch wearing a skirt'. Because it enhances that all-important sway, a lot of dancers wear scarves wrapped around their waist.

Q   Is there a dress code for slavercise?

A   'Cross-dressing' is encouraged apparently, whatever that means.

44

Shimmy yourself svelte

If your gym has just one dance class, then odds on it will be salsa. Here's why.

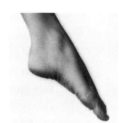

Salsa is smooth, sexy, but because it's based on relatively simple moves it can be learnt quite quickly (and then improved on forever).

As an aerobic workout salsa is low impact – and gets lower as you get better because the weight is kept on the ball of the foot in an elastic movement that cushions the step. It also works up more of a sweat than you might expect, particularly for beginners, so don't show up in your Sunday best. Men tend to have a harder time of it than women, which has the bonus that they get a more thorough workout (in style-defined exercise you tend to burn more calories the worse you are). The downside is that they sweat like beasts of burden and may be hard to entice back.

WHAT CAN I EXPECT?

Classes don't normally start with an exercise workout as such but rather with a refresher of the most basic steps. You may find these about as hard as walking, but if like me, you've got two left feet, you may end up with your brow furrowed and your legs all over the place for the first couple of lessons. Stick with it and it will come.

Here's an idea for you...

A lot of salsa clubs offer a deal combining a lesson and a night on the tiles. You show up for an hour or so before the club opens and have a refresher lesson in form or perhaps a new move or two. Because it's still early you then get to practice while the club is fairly empty, and most of the other people there will be the same dancers you met in the hour-long class. Not only have you already met but you are all there to learn so it makes finding partners much easier. By the time the club fills up you should be much less self-conscious and ready to show them what you're made of.

Moving on from there the initial moves are practised as individuals, but all classes rapidly move on to partner work. Don't worry if you didn't bring a partner. In a typical class everybody will be rotated to dance with everyone else. Salsa is pretty traditional in its sexual politics and the man is expected to lead. Since men tend to be in the minority, this means any bloke who shows his face will be guaranteed a warm reception, if only from women bored of learning male steps.

You're not really going to learn dancing from the pages of a book, but here are a couple of general pointers to make life easier when you're in the class.

In salsa you avoid having the weight on your heels – you always step on the ball of your foot whether going forwards or backwards. It keeps you lighter on your feet, and more mobile.

When things speed up, through confidence or a shift in the tempo, remember to make life easier (and more stylish) by making your steps smaller.

Even though the hip movement is often the most outstandingly slick aspect of the dance it is not a separate skill from the leg moves. Don't worry about practising your hip movement, focus on the steps and the hips will follow when you are relaxed enough to let the rhythm take over from your head.

Enjoy getting down to music in an atmosphere that's more about fun than exercise? Then take a look at IDEA 43, *Walk on the wild side*, for some more exotic alternatives.

Try another idea...

Relax your body and keep your eyes firmly fixed on your partner's face. Like they always say to people on window ledges, 'don't look down'. Start to think too much about your feet and they themselves will forget what comes next.

'Dancing is a perpendicular expression of a horizontal desire.'
GEORGE BERNARD SHAW.

Defining idea...

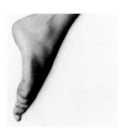
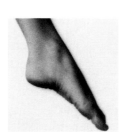
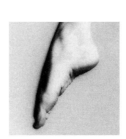
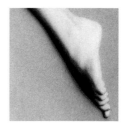

How did it go?

Q   What's the difference between a salsa class and Salsacise?

A   Salsacise is really aerobics moves set to a salsa beat. It will provide a decent cardio workout but won't help you too much when it comes to strutting your stuff on the dance floor.

Q   I'm a fairly regular salsa-goer but keep getting in a muddle when my partner leads and we try to perform any move where we let go, then take the other hand. Any ideas?

A   Keeping your arms up higher than waist height is a good discipline to get into right from the start since it helps with form and balance but also makes it much less likely that your arm will get stuck when you are 'wrapped in' by a partner. Missed hands in a move are often just down to practice but if your partner is taller than you, then holding them too low will make it harder to get it right.

Q   I found the first class OK but was back to square one when I returned for the next one while everybody else moved on. Am I destined to be left behind?

A   You may need to practice more between classes. The first class is really just about the basic steps. These should be burnt into your memory so find yourself doing them without thinking about it whenever the music starts (think the dole office scene in The Full Monty). Try practising them, however slowly, a couple of times a day – while you're getting dressed, in front of a mirror, in the bus queue, whenever.

45

In a spin

Fast, furious and fun, Spinning classes put you in a pack of fellow cyclists hurtling towards your fitness goals without having to take to the roads.

If stationary bikes leave you cold but you still like the idea of long lean legs and buttocks like balled up fists, then it's time to brave the Spinning studio.

Spinning is a trademark, by the way, so you may find it masquerading in your gym as RPM, or any one of a number of other aliases, but you can tell if you're in the right place the moment you swing a leg over the saddle. Start to turn the pedals and you'll realise that they are connected directly to a heavy flywheel. You spin, it spins. The trick is to remember that, unlike a bicycle, if you stop, it doesn't. To slow it down you have to press a knob that pushes a brake pad against the flywheel. To make life harder you have a control to increase the drag against the flywheel so it takes more effort to keep the pedals spinning around.

Here's an idea for you...

Spinning is pretty intensive so it pays to show up prepared. Of all the classes you've ever done this is the one where you'll die on your arse if you don't have a water bottle to hand. The latest spin bikes have a water holder on the handlebars or frame, the older ones aren't that far from the floor so just stop every now and again (remember to brake the flywheel before it yanks your foot off) and glug. While you're at it on the preparation, make sure you're dressed for the part – wicking tops and padded cycle shorts make sense (see also IDEA 1, *Looking the part*).

WHAT CAN I EXPECT?

Spinning classes start with some nice easy warm-up exercises to get you used to the feel of the bike, and to give you an idea of what's in store. There are three basic moves – sprints, climbs and jumps. Sprints are exactly what they sound like – the instructor encourages you to set a level of resistance and then burn away as fast as you can. Climbs mean a high level of resistance and standing on the pedals to keep it moving. Jumps mean short, sharp spells out of the saddle.

The instructor will encourage you to turn the resistance up and down depending on the 'road' ahead. Your gym will provide stomping music, perhaps darken the room, and maybe even put on a light show. The emphasis is on an all-singing all-dancing total absorption into the moment and the result is good, sweaty, cardio fun. If you're worried that the pace is likely to be too hectic for you, don't be. It's up to you how much you increase the resistance – your instructor's legs may spin like a washing machine but that doesn't mean you should follow suit straight away.

WHAT GOOD DOES IT DO?

Converts tend to see Spinning as the closest you can get to partying in the saddle. Even the less committed have to admit that the fierce calorie burn (up to double normal cycling on your own) plus the toning of hamstrings, calves, hips and abs adds up to quite a workout.

Enjoy spinning but prefer to practice on your own? A lot of the techniques and the strength required can be worked up on the stationary bike, see IDEAS 16 and 17, *On yer (stationary) bike I and II.*

Try another idea...

'When I see an adult on a bicycle, I do not despair of the future of the human race.'
H.G. WELLS

Defining idea...

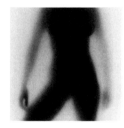

How did it go?

Q **I'm taking it as easy as I can but I'm still finding it really tough. My bum is black and blue! What am I doing wrong?**

A *One common mistake is to presume that if you keep the resistance really low, then you're in for an easy ride. In fact if you don't have enough resistance you may find it hard to control the bike, particularly for the sprints, and that means that you will bounce up and down more. Don't be afraid to up the resistance a bit.*

Q **I'm still getting a sore bum – in fact I think I get it worse because I'm not that naturally padded, if you follow.**

A *Go to a cycle or sports shop and ask for a gel saddle cover. It's a soft and squishy saddle-shaped thing you slip over the bike saddle to protect your nether bits. Enjoy.*

Q **I realise this is meant to be hard, but why do my knees and wrists ache?**

A *Sounds like your bike isn't properly adjusted for you. Remember these bikes adjust in two ways. The seat height goes up and down (it should be below your hip when you stand next to it, and your knee should still be very slightly bent at the bottom of the stroke). They also adjust at the front where the handlebars can move towards or away from you. If they're too far away, you'll stretch out and your weight will be on your wrists. Ask the instructor to help with the setup.*

46

Skipping

Small girls know that skipping is fun. Big, brutish boxers know that skipping is really tough. Somewhere in between those two extremes there's something for everyone.

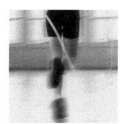

Skipping is a great way to increase stamina, improve co-ordination and tone muscles.

It's a huge calorie burner – for a 75 kg man think about 750 calories per hour. It gives much of the workout of running with far less impact. It doesn't require waiting in line for a treadmill either. It can be as complex or as simple as you like and while it takes a few sessions to get the basic skills it can be done by anybody. Indeed such are the joys of skipping for fitness that there is a regular rumour in the fitness industry that one of the big boys is about to introduce an aerobic class based on it.

Even if your gym doesn't have skipping ropes it has a place to skip and you can bring your own rope – they cost anywhere from a fiver to £20. If you are buying your own, look for one with a plastic rope and soft foam handles. Make sure that the handles will stay still in your hands while the rope turns. Superior leather ones are available but take a while to break in. Make sure you select one that's the right size for you – see below.

Try a boxer's workout. Skip for three minutes (the time of a round) then perform as many crunches as you can for a minute. Now skip for three minutes again, then perform as many press-ups as you can in a minute. Skip again for three minutes, then a minute of crunches. Repeat until you've worked out for half an hour. That should have worked out your speed, endurance, upper and lower body strength. The skipping means that your heartrate should remain significantly higher than usual even during the one-minute press up/crunch 'breaks' so it's a full half hour of cardio exercise.

SAFETY

I know, I know, safety issues may seen relative when you're talking about the favourite sport of schoolgirls but they probably don't have all that adult weight you're carrying.

Ensure the rope is the right size. When you're standing in the middle of it, each end should reach up to your armpits. If it's too long, then knot it. If it's too short, then get another one.

Make sure you're wearing shoes meant for bounding up and down – that means cross-trainers or basketball shoes but not running shoes. Women: is your bra up to this?

STRETCH BEFORE YOU SKIP.

Try to avoid skipping on concrete or a wooden floor that's laid directly on concrete. Your gym has exercise mats – use one. In fact use two or three if they're spare, or better yet skip on the thick mat area that's sometimes laid out for stretching. Try not to skip on those trying to stretch. You can't leg it like you could in fourth form.

GETTING GOING

The basic skip step is the pogo with both feet bouncing off the ground together as the rope passes under. Try to keep the weight nice and light on the balls of your feet and make sure you've got good rhythm before trying to increase the speed or you'll wind up as a red-faced tangle of rope and blasphemy.

When you start out, aim for short bursts of 20 seconds or so before taking a brief break (a good time to stretch) and then repeating. Build it up slowly until you can leave out the breaks and skip for five minutes or more straight. Once you're there it's time to get fancy with the footwork. Simple variations are hopping on one foot and swapping over, or alternating between heel and toe landings. As you get better try the following:

Side swing – Swing the rope to the side of you so it taps the ground as it passes by the outside of your leg. Next jump is normal through the rope, then swing the rope to the other side past the other leg. Doesn't sound much but done at speed you become a blur of rope with a satisfying tapping sound.

Cross jumps – As the rope comes over your head, cross your hands and jump through the rope. You'll have to keep your hands crossed as you bring them back up your body and uncross as the rope comes over your head again or else you're going to smack yourself silly.

Skipping is a true plyometric exercise, to learn more about that turn to IDEA 22, *Explode into action.*

Try another idea...

**Jelly on a plate,
Jelly on a plate,
Wibble wobble, wibble wobble
Jelly on a plate.**
Traditional rhyme

Defining idea...

How did it go?

Q **It's great but I get really tired and my calves are killing me. I know this is meant to be a workout but should it be this hard?**

A *Sounds like you may be jumping too high off the ground. Good skippers only come 2.5 cm (1 inch) off the ground with each jump. Jumping higher uses more calories but stretches your calves more and increases the impact.*

Q **I'm trying a trick or two here but finding it frustrating as I keep wrapping the rope around myself. How can I avoid self-strangulation?**

A *Try tricks, or indeed anything new, without the rope. At first this will seem strange but it's a great way of learning the rhythm of a move without constantly thwacking yourself in the legs.*

Q **How often should I skip?**

A *In the beginning aim to skip just two or three times a week for a total of five to ten minutes at a time because you'll feel it in your lower arms and calves. Build up as you feel more confident.*

47

Hi Lo and BodyAttack

Lots of impact, lots of leaping, breathlessness and 'the burn' are what draw people to these two different approaches to aerobics.

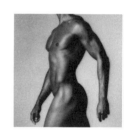

BodyAttack versus Hi Lo — evolution in action

Twenty years ago any gym that aimed to encourage both sexes would have had a class called aerobics where the emphasis was on loud music, high-energy dance moves and slightly more whooping than you get in the free weights room. These days the last remnants of that approach can be found in the likes of BodyAttack and Hi Lo which both work on the same principle (loud music, lots of calorie expenditure) but with a difference that says a lot about the way the gym business is going. The benefits of both are improved circulation, stronger heart and lungs, lower cholesterol and increased bone density (providing you don't break any in the process).

BodyAttack follows the tried and trusted format of other Les Mills exercise routines (such as BodyPump and RPM) which means that you warm up and then go through a certain number of basic routines followed by a brief abs and cool-down finale. The music is changed every few months to keep it fresh but the exercises remain the same. Once you've been to one you can walk into a BodyAttack class in Beirut or Bangor and immediately know what comes next. In fact what comes next is a mix of work on the spot, forward backward advances and movements circling the

201

Here's an idea for you...

Not all Hi Lo classes are the same. If your gym does a class called Cardio Low or Cardio Jam you may want to try that as a gentle introduction to the glories of Hi Lo. If not, then find the instructor and explain your choreographic limitations – he'll tell you which of the weekly classes tends to be the most hardcore. If your gym does both, then BodyAttack is an easier place to start out than some of the Hi Lo classes for aerobics addicts.

studio. There's a huge amount of hopping involved which in itself is very high impact and not recommended for those with joint problems or weak shins. Good cross-trainers are essential. BodyAttack's choreography is not challenging – even the most clodhopping will pick it up straight away – which leaves the emphasis firmly on working up a sweat.

If you're used to the Les Mills approach to courses (such as BodyPump, RPM or BodyAttack), then Hi Lo will come as a bit of a surprise. Hi Lo is very much open for interpretation and will vary wildly from one gym to the next and one instructor to another.

A normal programme would kick off with 5–10 minutes of warm-up, then a peak of 20–30 minutes of target heart range dancing, followed by 20 minutes of body sculpting (a muscle-stretching floor session) and ending with cool-down and stretches.

The Hi Lo refers to the mix of high and low intensity moves which is a coded warning that the class may get a bit frenetic (lots of leaping). It also usually means that there will be some challenging choreography with the instructors allowed to get as creative as they choose. In practice that means that classes will be a lot more fun for regulars, but can be off-putting for newcomers unless they're particularly good at picking up new moves. Definitely the place to be for girl band wannabes, not necessarily so right for hairy truckers with two left feet.

Depending on the nature of the group you find yourself in you may also find that part of the requirement of either of the above is to make more whooping noises than a coach load of gibbons arriving at Disneyland. It's all part of the fun.

Try another idea...

Music, choreography, impact and high calorie burn are also the hallmarks of step classes – try IDEA 15, *Stepping up a gear.*

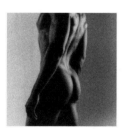

Defining idea...

'The word "aerobics" came about when the gym instructors got together and said: if we're going to charge $10 an hour, we can't call it Jumping Up And Down.'
RITA RUDNER, US comedian

How did it go?

Q   I'm wearing proper cross-trainers. Why am I still getting pain in my ankles?

A   *Studies show that the forces on your feet in aerobics classes can be up to six times that of gravity. If you have pronounced pronation or supination (see IDEA 1, Looking the part) you may need stabilising shoes to counterbalance that effect.*

Q   I'd love to keep up but I can't for the life of me. Help!

A   *Try practising at home. Draw the curtains, fire up the DVD or video and do your own sessions. The way aerobics choreography works means that a lot of moves are really chains of quite simple basic steps which you will find on popular videos/DVDs. Your instructor may be able to recommend the best ones to watch to keep up with a particular class.*

Q   The instructor is talking gibberish. What's a grapevine?

A   *Aerobics does have its own vocabulary – take a look at the Turnstep dictionary of moves (www.turnstep.com/moves) which details what they all are and has animations to help explain.*

48

Vicious circuits

A complete body workout in the space of a single lunch hour? That, in a nutshell, is the appeal of circuit training.

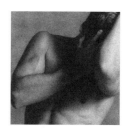

It's theoretically possible to set up a circuit training session on your own using the gym equipment.

Just as you are about to move on to another piece of equipment, however, Sod's Law says that someone will start using it for you. In some parts of the world gyms take circuit training so seriously that they have steps, stations and weight training machines permanently set up for circuits and nothing else. Lights and beepers time down each set and warn you to move on to the next one. That's relatively rare in the UK, which is not altogether a bad thing since the beeper can drive everyone else up the wall. If your gym does have an area set aside for circuits, then great, but you'll probably end up doing them as a one-hour class, often in the lunchtime slot.

That's because they really are a great way to pack in a lot of variety and hard work in a short period of time.

Variety – because a circuit can consists of a dozen or more different exercises which mix and match strength and cardio workouts.

Hard work – because knowing that you only have a couple of minutes on each one makes it easier to go for it for that period. A well-organised circuit alternates

205

At first you'll probably find circuit training sessions quite enough to leave you exhausted, but as you get better you may want to make individual stations more demanding. The circuit approach leaves you plenty of leeway to do just that. For press-ups, try putting your feet (or shins if that's too tough) up on a bench, or rest one foot on the heel of the other to focus a little more on balance. Other variations include a wide stance where your hands are more than shoulder-width apart (works the arms less and the chest more), or a narrow stance where your hands are as close together as you can bear (which focuses on the triceps). For a very different feel, try off-setting your hands so one is a bit forward and the other a bit behind the line of your shoulders. This creates an instability that should get to work on those stabilising muscles in your back, as well as your abs and obliques.

between strength and cardio stations, or between upper and lower body so that each station functions as an 'active rest' period for the last. Since stations change according to the whim of the instructors you may also find yourself trying exercises you wouldn't normally do. See it as a kind of exercise speed dating.

For crunches, try to perform the crunch while also keeping both legs off the ground to work the lower abs a little. Since circuit training often pairs people off to work the stations together, how about going with a friend and indulging in a little competition about who can do the greatest number of reps during the session?

WHAT CAN I EXPECT?

Typical moves to include in a circuit are squats and step-ups (using a bench) to work the lower body, plus crunches and bicycle kicks for the abs. Favourites include press-ups to work the chest and some explosive work such as jumping jacks (star jumps) or burpees, where you start in the press-up position but work by shooting your legs back and forth to bring your knees to your elbows. Shuttle runs and skipping are commonly included to keep the heartrate up and add an endurance factor to the circuit. Some dumbbell or barbell work may be included to work specific muscles but the usual rule of thumb is that circuit training is about compound exercises that work as many muscles as possible at once. Where there are weights they will be light and the aim is to do as many repetitions as you can manage during the session. Session lengths may vary but 60 seconds is common and the overall goal is maximum fitness result in minimum time – something we can all relate to.

Try another idea...

If you're interested in high energy mixing and matching read a little more about interval training in IDEA 37, *The cardio cocktail.*

Defining idea...

'Leave all the afternoon for exercise and recreation, which are as necessary as reading. I will rather say more necessary because health is worth more than learning.'
THOMAS JEFFERSON, a man with more time for exercise than most of us.

How did it go?

Q **I am aiming to do my own circuit in the gym using the equipment provided. Is the one minute per station rule the best way?**

A *Depends on your goals and your level of workout. It's often harder to keep up the tempo on your own so you may want to try the following. Complete your set of 10 or 12 different exercises for a minute each, then take a 'rest' break of cardio work (skipping, running, cycling, etc.) for 8–10 minutes before launching into the next circuit. The idea is that it helps maintain the aerobic pace of the session and keep your heart working harder.*

Q **Will running shoes do for circuits?**

A *Not ideally, no. While it's hard to second-guess what your instructor is going to include in a circuit, the smart money is on a fair amount of jumping. Running shoes won't provide the cushioning for that, or protect your ankle from sudden changes in direction (as you get in shuttle runs). If you're really going to go for it then invest in a pair of decent cross-trainers.*

Q **We do a lot of bench dips in circuit class. Any way I can train for that?**

A *Try doing bench dips but with elevated feet. If you have your feet on one bench, and your hands behind you on another, then it is far harder to dip than with your feet on the floor. Ensure you drop down so that your upper arm is parallel to the floor and your elbow is bent at a 90 degree angle.*

49

Squat yet bijoux

Squats power up your thighs, hips, calves and buttocks, and using free weights they also work your back, abs and obliques. With so many benefits from one simple move it seems a shame to leave them to powerlifters.

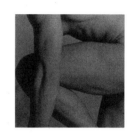

Squats train your body in balance, they strengthen the stabilisers and tone the thighs and buttocks.

They can increase your flexibility and range of movement, they provide the driving force for runners and jumpers, and with attention to form they can protect your back from the wear and tear of daily life. So much from so little. Yet most of us shy away from squats in the belief that they are best left to vast pumped-up East Europeans.

There are lots of reasons why people shy away from squats but the main ones are:

■ Fear of provoking back trouble.
■ Fear of ending up looking like a powerlifter.
■ They're hard.
■ They are the opposite of glamour – even the name is ugly.

Here's an idea for you...

Because balancing brings in so many other muscles to help lift weight, it's great exercise to introduce a certain amount of controlled instability. By doing a one-legged squat you will call on all the stabilising muscles of your joints and your mid-section. Start off with legs slightly bent, shoulder-width apart and with a single dumbbell held in both hands on the top of your chest so your chin can rest on it. Now lift your right foot up so your calf is parallel to the floor. Now bend your left leg at the knee and slowly lower your body. If you can make it to the point where your thigh is parallel to the floor bravo, if not then stop before then. Smoothly straighten your leg to return to the starting position. This is undoubtedly a tough one, and you should start with a lighter weight than usually, not least because if you overbalance the first few times you may drop it.

OK, the last point is a fair cop, but the whole point of the gym thing is how you look outside, not while you're in there. As for the others they all seem to presume that you're going to squat with weights the size of car wheels on each end of the bar. The basic squat can be done with nothing more than your own bodyweight if you prefer, and adding a barbell (or dumbbells – see IDEA 40, *Getting smart with dumbbells II*) should be done when you're ready. Small weights and good form will do far more for you than large weights hefted around with scant consideration for your back.

SQUATS WITH YOUR OWN BODYWEIGHT

Start off with your feet shoulder-width apart and your legs very lightly bent at the knee. Breathe in and pull your shoulders back a little so that your spine assumes its natural curve in your lower back. You may find it more comfortable to open the stance slightly by pointing your toes outwards. Just remember that your knees must move in the same axis as your feet, so toes outwards means your knees move outwards too – otherwise you'll set up a turning force and risk strain.

With your arms out straight in front of you like a sleepwalker, bend your knees and ease yourself down as if sitting into an armchair. The lift is done by straightening those knees and driving down through the legs and heels. If you find yourself lifting onto the balls of your feet, then you are unbalanced forwards. Keep the whole sole of your foot firmly planted on the floor.

If you want to try your squat technique where an instructor can watch you, then go to a BodyPump class where you'll find that squats are the first session after the warm-up. See IDEA 33, *Pump that body*.

Try another idea...

Once you're comfortable doing squats without weight, try the broomstick (your gym may have a nicer name for it but you'll recognise it as a broomstick) held across the back of your shoulders. Watch yourself in the mirror as you squat to ensure your head and neck are straight up and the natural curve of your spine isn't exaggerated as you work. Happy with three sets of 12 reps with the stick? Time to move to the barbell.

'The back squat is king for building size and strength...it should be regarded as the most useful free-weights exercise.'
HARDGAINER MAGAZINE, the self-declared 'bastion of no-nonsense drug-free training'.

Defining idea...

How did it go?

Q **Looking in the mirror I realise that as I squat my knees turn inwards slightly. Is this normal?**

A *It's not ideal and could either mean poor technique or a weakness in your hip abductors. Does your gym have those rubber exercise bands to hand? If so, try looping one around your knees so that you have to have them slightly apart to stop the band from slipping off (if the band is big you may have to knot it to make it the right size). Now do your squats without letting the band drop as you bend.*

Q **Why do squats with the barbell hurt my neck?**

A *You can wrap a sweat towel around the bar, but check for a moment if you are resting the bar in the right place. Don't rest it on one of the knobbly bits that stick out at the bottom of your neck – those are vertebrae and we're trying to work muscle not spine. Instead hunch your shoulders up and reach back with one hand to feel the top of your back. You should be able to feel the trapezius muscles and the 'shelf' formed by the top of the muscle right across your shoulders. Aim to rest the bar there.*

Q **Why do my heels rise off the floor as I lower into the squat?**

A *You may have tight calves. In the short term make sure you pause at the bottom of the squat and place your heels firmly on the floor before driving upwards. In the long term you should try calf stretches. Try standing on a step with both feet together, balls of the feet on the edge of the step, heels out in space. Now pivoting with the middle of your sole on the edge of the step, lower one heel at a time and feel the stretch.*

50

Ab attack

Fab abs are top of the wishlist for men and women alike.

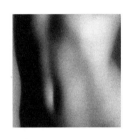

So why do so many people just stick to the basic crunch and hope for the best?

Get real – Your abs won't really show until you've burnt off the fat that's covering them and for men that means getting down to around 15 per cent body fat or lower, 25 per cent or lower for women (see IDEA 52, *Are we nearly there yet?*, for more).

There's no such thing as spot reduction, so you can't burn fat off one place on your body just by working that area, which means that real abs work is done on the treadmills and aerobics studio floor. What you can do, however, is tone up those muscles to help reduce back strain, improve balance and prepare for the day when, butterfly-like, they emerge from your wobbly chrysalis. To help with that it's best to start with a little bit of anatomy.

Instructors in ab attack classes (or legs, bums, tums – whatever your gym calls them) often refer to upper and lower abs. This is slightly misleading since they're really referring to the upper and lower sections of the same muscle, the rectus abdominis (the celebrated six-pack). The classic crunch works the upper abs; leg lifts, heel taps and bicycle kicking work the lower. To complete the picture you should also work the obliques down the sides which pull your waist in and help shape the stomach, and the transversus which lies deep beneath the abs and gives strength and shape to your whole midsection.

What most of us want when it comes to abs is tone rather than size or strength and a lot of that comes not from how developed the muscle is, but how taut it is. The key to tautness is keeping those abs contracted throughout exercises, and indeed throughout the day. One approach is to tie a piece of string around your waist (under your clothes of course) so that if you let your belly out it will touch the string. The idea is that it becomes a subconscious reminder and whenever your tum touches string it makes you pull it in, effectively exercising your abs all day long.

Ever wondered why you do abs exercises at the end of combination workout classes (like BodyPump or Hi Lo)? The idea is that if you did them before you'd run the risk of working out with tired ab muscles which could lead to bad posture. That's a lesson worth taking into your own individual workouts too, especially if you are going to be doing anything like squats, lunges or free weights where proper posture is what you rely on to prevent putting your back out.

Stomach muscles don't have the ability to bulk up like other muscles so don't worry about working them too hard. You can work them too often though – light abs work can be done daily but after a hard session they need a day off just like any other part of your body if they are to repair damage and grow stronger. Remember that it's while you rest that you get stronger.

Good exercises to focus on if you only have a few minutes to spare for the mat are twisting oblique raises and bicycling. These together hit pretty much the whole midsection.

For twisting oblique raises, adopt the normal crunch position on your back with legs bent. Now drop both knees to one side and keep them there as you lift the shoulders off the floor. Don't come up too high. After about 30 degrees your hip flexors take up the movement and the effort on your abs and obliques is reduced. Take it nice and slow.

For bicycling, start on your back with your legs straight and raise them both a few inches off the ground. Don't rest either leg back on the ground for the duration of the exercise. With hands on ears lift your shoulders off the ground in classic crunch style. You should bend your left knee and bring it up towards your chest, simultaneously twisting so your right elbow reaches down to meet it. Alternate elbows/knees and keep the whole movement as slow and smooth as you can.

The best exercises for reaching the deep transversus muscle are those aimed at core stability. Try varying your abs routine by taking a look at Pilates (IDEA 36, *Piling on the Pilates*) or body core classes (IDEA 30, *Hard core*). If you think that you lack strength in your mid section and aren't getting anywhere with standard abs exercises, then try IDEA 19, *Roman revenge*, or IDEA 20, *Hanging around*, for the short, sharp, shock treatment.

Try another idea...

'Belly gonna get ya.'
FROM A RUNNING SHOES AD

Defining idea...

How did
it go?

Q **How come I get neck ache when I lift my shoulder off the floor?**

A *It could be that your neck muscles aren't strong enough to take the weight – don't hesitate to support the back of your skull with your hand. It could also be a question of posture. Don't dig your chin into your chest as you lift up since this will stretch your neck. Keep an imaginary tennis ball between your chin and the top of your chest to ensure the correct posture.*

Q **Although I'm trying to pull my stomach in, my whole midsection is actually curving upwards when I lie on my back. Is that right?**

A *Depending on the exercise you're doing at the time (check with your instructor) it's normal to tilt the pelvis forward which flattens your stomach into the floor. Squeezing your buttocks together and tilting the pelvis forward is itself a pretty effective move for the lower abs.*

Q **I've always done alternate single leg lifts for my lower abs and now I'm told they're useless. Is that true?**

A *Useless is a strong word but studies suggest that while double leg lifts work the lower abs, single leg lifts with the other leg supported on the floor only really work the psoas muscle (deep inside your pelvic girdle) which won't make any visible difference.*

51

Cable Manners

Cable stations aren't just something you find on skiing holidays. Cable and pulley systems offer the safety of machines with the flexibility of free weights.

Cable stations consist of a stack of weights hooked up to a handle by means of a cable which runs over a pulley.

The one you've most likely used is a lat pull down – you sit down and pull a wide grip handle down towards you. Look around the weights room and there is probably a cable station at some point with cables coming off high pulleys (so you pull down) or low pulleys (so you pull up). There may even be a crossover station, a contraption where you stand between two sets of weights attached to pulleys and cables with handles. Given that there seem to be dedicated machines for biceps, triceps, chest, shoulders and earlobe exercises, you might wonder what the point of cable stations is. In which case you may be surprised to learn that legions of strength trainers absolutely swear by them. Pulley power is king.

Cable/pulley weights give you a lot of freedom of movement (as you'll see from these sample exercises) which lets you work muscles differently. Take a look at the crossover exercises and try and figure out how you would do those with free weights. Cable weights also apply pressure evenly throughout, which makes your muscles work through their entire range of movement. In a lot of free weights moves there is a point where balance means that your muscle is actually resting –

One of the handle types you may see lying around near the base of the station is a rope handle. Try this for pull down/up exercises and you'll find that it makes them much harder because it is more difficult to grip and so works the forearm and wrist muscles.

such as the top point of a curl before your arm starts lowering again. With a cable, however, the thing is always pulling against you for as long as you have it in your hand. The little scamps keep working until you put them down. With that in mind, try a few of the following.

CABLE CROSSOVERS

You'll need a crossover station here, with a set of weights/pulley/cable on each side of you. Set the cable to a low pulley on each side and with a handle in each hand start with your arms out away from your sides. Now bring your hands together until your wrists cross in front of your face, then slowly return to the starting position. That works shoulders and pecs. For variety, set up the stations so the cables come off the high pulleys and start with your arms out wide and high (crucifix position) before pulling down until your wrists cross in front of your groin like a footie player waiting to block a direct free kick. If you only have one cable station in the gym, then you can perform either of these moves with just one arm at a time.

STANDING CURL

Stand in front of a low pulley holding the bar in both hands in front of your groin, palms turned away from you. Without moving your shoulders or upper arms, bend your elbows and curl the weight up to your shoulders. Great for biceps.

STANDING SHRUG

Stand as for the curl but holding the bar with palms turned towards you. Keeping your hands straight, lift the bar by shrugging your shoulders up towards your ears. Works the trapezius muscles of your upper back.

If you like working with weights but not the free weights, then check out the Gravitron machine in IDEA 23, *Getting groovy with the Gravitron.*

Try another idea…

SEATED TRICEPS EXTENSION

Pull a bench over to the low pulley and sit down with your back to the machine. Hold the bar in both hands and pull up so that your arms are straight up above your head. Without moving your upper arms, bend your elbows so your forearms go back and your hands end up behind your head with your forearms parallel to the floor. Straighten your arms again.

PUSH-DOWN TRICEPS EXTENSION

Stand facing a high pulley, holding the bar with both hands and your arms straight down so the bar is pulled down to your groin. Bend your elbows so your hands and forearms rise to horizontal in front of you. Straighten your arms again and push the weight back down.

'The last three or four reps is what makes the muscle grow. This area of pain divides the champion from someone else who is not a champion.'
ARNOLD SCHWARZENEGGER

Defining idea…

How did it go?

Q   Low pulley, high pulley – how does that work then?

A   *Look closely at the pulley system and you'll see that where there is both a low and a high pulley, it's usually possible to unclip a part of the cable so that it comes off one or the other. Most machines are designed to work in either position and it's down to you to set them up one way or the other. If in doubt, drag a gym instructor over and insist she shows you how.*

Q   Why is there a funny looking handle on this one?

A   *It's not just the pulley height that can be adjusted. The handles on pulley systems can be clipped on or off and swapped with a choice of rope handles, wide grip bars or doubled handed grips (like the handles on swing doors) for rowing motions.*

52

Are we nearly there yet? Measuring your progress

If you don't know what you're trying to achieve, how will you know if you've done it? Let's look at some ways to monitor progress.

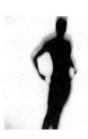

Ask most people why they go to the gym and they'll say that they want to 'lose weight and tone up' or 'get fitter'.

All of which are admirable goals, but a little vague. Without a clear sense of progress it's easy to lose motivation, and vague goals make it hard to measure solid achievements. So here are few ideas for measuring your own progress.

WEIGHT

Chances are that you don't really want to lose weight. What you want to lose is fat, and the scales may not be telling you the whole truth. Muscle is denser than fat so it is entirely possible that exercise will successfully swap fat for muscle but leave your weight unchanged. So if the scales alone won't tell you the good news, what can you do?

The best thing to do is stop thinking weight and start thinking about how much of that weight is fat which is surplus to requirements. That means measuring your body

Here's an idea for you...

BMI isn't perfect but with a bit of mental agility (or a calculator) you can work it out yourself. To find your BMI take your height in metres and multiply the figure by itself. Then take your weight in kilograms and divide the weight by the height squared.

For a man 1.8 m tall and weighing 80 kg that calculation would be
Height times itself
(1.8 x 1.8 = 3.24)
Weight divided by that
(80/3.24 = 24.69)
For men the normal score is 21–26, so this is normal.
For women that range is 18–23.

fat percentage. There are several ways to do this. Calipers can be used to measure folds of flesh at various points around your body where fat is stored and a calculation can be done on the basis of your age and gender to come up with a percentage. Some gyms will do this for you. But it's considerably easier and much quicker to use an electric body fat monitor. These are much like scales except that they pass a tiny electrical current (you don't feel a thing, honest) through your body. Fat, muscle and water all conduct electricity at different speeds and so given a bit of information about your height, weight, age and sex, the monitor can produce a figure for your body fat percentage. If your gym doesn't have one of these devices you can get home monitors that double up as scales. It's not an infallible system as the amount of water in your body changes over the day and can give different readings at different times. Nonetheless if used properly a body fat monitor gives a more accurate reading than weight alone. According to the World Health Organization, the healthy range for men aged 20–39 is from 8–20 per cent body fat, for women it is 21–33. Seeing your body fat figure coming down is one of the most motivating factors of going to the gym.

BMI – Another comparative figure that's often used is body mass index, or BMI. BMI is the relationship of your weight to your height. There are plenty of BMI calculators available online, including one at the BBC's website (www.bbc.co.uk/health).

BMI is criticised by some because it doesn't take into account your build or muscle mass. A 90 kg couch potato and a 90 kg Royal Marine are both treated equally. Nonetheless it is a better guide to your shape than weight alone and can give you an idea of your target range of weight.

If you like the idea of measuring your progress against a set of familiar exercises, then try circuit training – see IDEA 48, *Vicious circuits.*

Try another idea...

STRENGTH

The US military physical fitness test standard is to be able to complete at least 40 press-ups in less than two minutes, at least 50 sit-ups in under two minutes, do six pull ups (chins), and run 2.5 km in under 12 minutes. That's for fully trained professional soldiers, mind you, not raw recruits.

For those of us not aiming to compete with GI Joes/Janes here are a few more reasonable figures.

Men – just try doing as many press-ups as you can in one go. If you're under 30 and you can do 45 or more, then you're right up there; 35–44 is average. If you're 30–40, then over 35 press-ups is impressive, and 25–34 is average. For 40–50 year olds those figures read 30 or more for tough guys, 20–29 for average Joes. For **women** – (using knees on the ground press-ups) that figure for under thirties is 34 press-ups or more for the superfit, 17–33 for the averagely fit. For women aged 30–40, then 25 press-ups secures your place in the superfit slot, and 12–24 sees you in the average group. Women aged 40–50 who can do 20 press-ups or more should be letting people know about it, and those capable of 8–19 are safe in the knowledge that they make the grade.

'The limits of the possible can only be defined by going beyond them into the impossible.'
ARTHUR C. CLARKE

Defining idea...

223

How did it go?

Q I'm not good at press-ups but believe I am strong in the lower body. Is there a test for that?

A *Yes, try 'the chair'. Stand with your back against a wall and feet shoulder-width apart. Now slide down the wall until your thighs are parallel to the ground as if you were sitting on an invisible chair. See how long you can hold the position. Over a minute, excellent; 41–60 seconds, good; 31–40 seconds, average.*

Q My BMI is through the roof but I don't believe I am that out of shape. What's going on?

A *You may not be; it's a very rough guideline. See a high BMI as an indicator that it's time to get your body fat percentage measured – ask at your gym.*

Q Is there a swimming test for fitness?

A *Not a general fitness test no, although if you want to compare yourself with GI Joe, then being able to swim 500 m in 12 minutes would mean you can keep up with Uncle Sam's swimmers.*

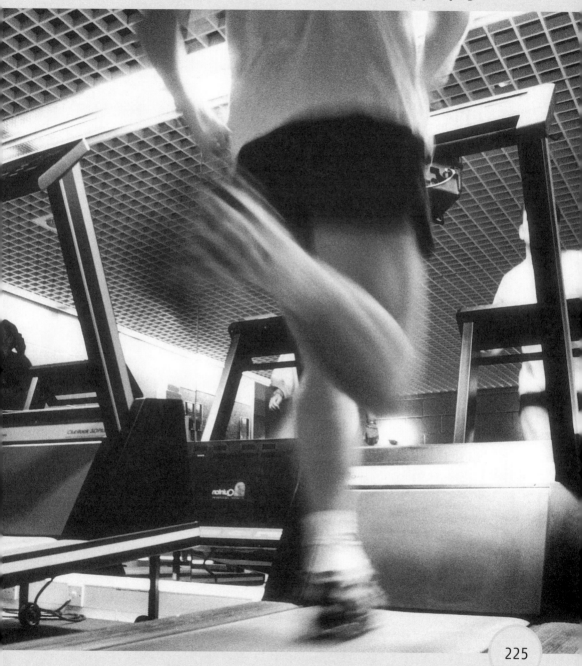

The end...

Or is it a new beginning? We hope that the ideas in this book will have inspired you to try new things and put the spice back into your gym life. You should be well on your way to a fitter, firmer you, with a fresh spring in your step and a fistful of goals.

You're mean, you're motivated and you don't care who the hell knows it.

So why not let *us* know about it? Tell us how you got on. What did it for you – what helped you punch through the plateaux and beat the boredom? Maybe you've got some tips of your own you want to share (see next page). If you liked this book you may find we have more brilliant ideas for other areas that could help change your life for the better.

You'll find Steve Shipside and the rest of the Infinite Ideas crew waiting for you online at www.infideas.com.

Or if you prefer to write, then send your letters to:
Win at the Gym
The Infinite Ideas Company Ltd
Belsyre Court, 57 Woodstock Road, Oxford OX2 6JH, United Kingdom

We want to know what you think, because we're all working on making our lives better too. Give us your feedback and you could win a copy of another *52 Brilliant Ideas* book of your choice. Or maybe get a crack at writing your own.

Good luck. Be brilliant.

Offer one

CASH IN YOUR IDEAS

We hope you enjoy this book. We hope it inspires, amuses, educates and entertains you. But we don't assume that you're a novice, or that this is the first book that you've bought on the subject. You've got ideas of your own. Maybe our author has missed an idea that you use successfully. If so, why not send it to info@infideas.com, and if we like it we'll post it on our bulletin board. Better still, if your idea makes it into print we'll send you £50 and you'll be fully credited so that everyone knows you've had another Brilliant Idea.

Offer two

HOW COULD YOU REFUSE?

Amazing discounts on bulk quantities of Infinite Ideas books are available to corporations, professional associations and other organizations.

For details call us on:
+44 (0)1865 292045
fax: +44 (0)1865 292001
or e-mail: info@infideas.com

Where it's at...